Instant Caregiver Kit

Instant Caregiver Kit

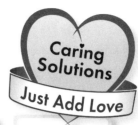

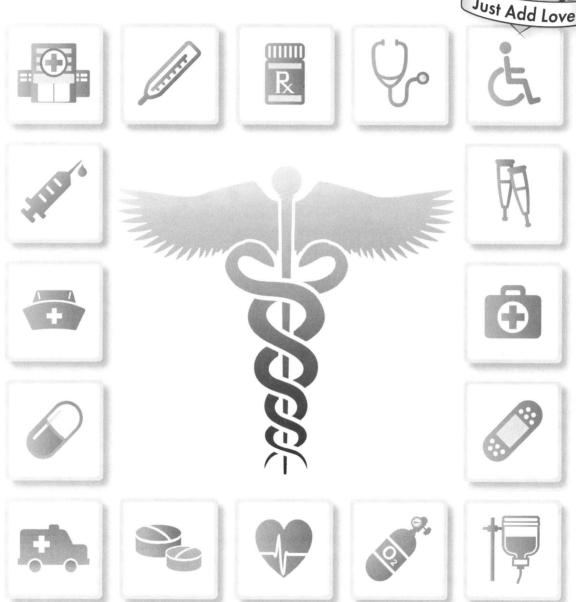

By Rebecca Sharp Colmer and Regina Caswell, RN
EKLEKTIKA PRESS
Chelsea, Michigan

©2009 by Rebecca Sharp Colmer

First Printing

EKLEKTIKA Press
P. O. Box 157
Chelsea, MI 48118

All rights reserved. No part of this book may be reproduced or transmitted in any form by any means, electronic or mechanical, including photocopying, recording, or by any information storage and retrieval system without written permission from the author.

All trademarks mentioned in this book are the property of their representative owners. Any third-party Web sites mentioned in this book are not sponsored or endorsed by EKLEKTIKA, Inc. or Me and My Caregivers, Inc.

Copyright 2009 by Rebecca Sharp Colmer

ISBN-13: 978-0-9765465-8-0

Printed in the United States of America

Table of Contents

Introduction 8

Part 1: Frequently Asked Questions 9

About Caregivers and Caregiving 10
About Care-Receivers 14
Health Issues Associated with Aging 16
First Aid/Emergencies/CPR 19
Getting Ready 22
Communication and Decision Making 22
Assembling the Care Team 24
Preparing the Home 39
Getting Through the Day 44
Managing Feelings 44
Taking Care of Yourself While Caregiving 47

Part 2: Forms 49

How To Use The Forms 50
Getting Started Checklist 53
Budget Worksheet 54
Valuable Records Checklist 55
General Care Evaluation 59
Personal Care Checklist 60
Release of Information and Consent Form 62
In Case of Emergency 63
Emergency Wallet Card 64
Living Will Directive 65
Health Care Proxy and Durable Power of Attorney for Health Care 67
Emergency Medical Services Prehospital Do Not Resuscitate (Dnr) Form 69
Personal Information 70
Care Team Contact Information 71
My Health Now 72
My Past Health History 73
My Daily Living Routine and Activities 74
Leisure and Recreational Activities 76
Calendar 77
Questions For The Doctor 78
Lab Tests, X-Rays & Hospital Visits 79
Reminders/Shopping List 80
My Medications 81
Daily Logs 82
Respite Caregiver Checklist 84
End-of-Life Issues Checklist 86

Part 3: Extras 87

101 Tips 88
Resources 92
Glossary 95
Alzheimer's Disease and Caregiving 101
Bonus: Caring for the Caregiver 102

Acknowledgments

Thank you to the many care-receivers and caregivers who shared their hearts with me. To each and every one of you, I am grateful.

A special thank you to Ginny Wood-Bailey, LMSW.

As always, a special thank you to my husband, Flip Colmer, an invaluable source of love, support and understanding.

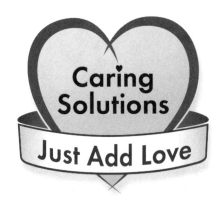

Disclaimer

Every effort has been made to make this book as complete as possible and as accurate as possible. However, there may be mistakes both typographical and in content. Therefore, this text should be used as a general guide and not the ultimate source of information.

The medical and legal information and procedures contained in this book are not intended as a substitute for consulting your physician or attorney. Because there is always some risk involved, the publisher and author are not responsible for any adverse effects or consequences resulting from the use of any suggestions, preparations, or procedures in this book. Please do not use the book is you are unwilling to assume the risk.

LIMIT OF LIABILITY/DISCLAIMER OF WARRANTY: THE PUBLISHER AND THE AUTHOR MAKE NO REPRESENTATIONS OR WARRANTIES WITH RESPECT TO THE ACCURACY OR COMPLETENESS OF THE CONTENTS OF THIS WORK AND SPECIFICALLY DISCLAIM ALL WARRANTIES, INCLUDING WITHOUT LIMITATION WARRANTIES OF FITNESS FOR A PARTICULAR PURPOSE. NO WARRANTY MAY BE CREATED OR EXTENDED BY SALES OR PROMOTIONAL MATERIALS. THE ADVICE AND STRATEGIES CONTAINED HEREIN MAY NOT BE SUITABLE FOR EVERY SITUATION. THIS WORK IS SOLD WITH THE UNDERSTANDING THAT THE PUBLISHER IS NOT ENGAGED IN RENDERING LEGAL, MEDICAL, ACCOUNTING, OR OTHER PROFESSIONAL SERVICES. IF PROFESSIONAL ASSISTANCE IS REQUIRED, THE SERVICES OF A COMPETENT PROFESSIONAL PERSON SHOULD BE SOUGHT. NEITHER THE PUBLISHER NOR THE AUTHOR SHALL BE LIABLE FOR DAMAGES ARISING HEREFROM. THE FACT THAT AN ORGANIZATION OR WEB SITE IS REFERRED TO IN THIS WORK AS A CITATION AND/OR POTENTIAL SOURCE OF FURTHER INFORMATION DOES NOT MEAN THAT THE AUTHOR OR THE PUBLISHER ENDORSES THE INFORMATION THE ORGANIZATION OR WEB SITE MAY PROVIDE OR RECOMMENDATIONS IT MAY MAKE. FURTHER, READERS SHOULD BE AWARE THAT INTERNET WEB SITES LISTED IN THIS WORK MAY HAVE CHANGED OR DISAPPEARED BETWEEN WHEN IT WAS WRITTEN AND WHEN IT IS READ. NEITHER THE PUBLISHER NOR AUTHOR SHALL BE LIABLE FOR ANY LOSS OF PROFIT OR ANY OTHER COMMERCIAL DAMAGES, INCLUDING BUT NOT LIMITED TO SPECIAL, INCIDENTAL, CONSEQUENTIAL, OR OTHER DAMAGES. THE AUTHOR AND PUBLISHER SPECIFICALLY DISCLAIM ANY LIABILITY, LOSS, OR RISK, PERSONAL OR OTHERWISE, WHICH IS INCURRED AS A CONSEQUENCE, DIRECTLY OR INDIRECTLY, OF THE USE AND APPLICATION OF ANY OF THE CONTENTS OF THIS BOOK.

Introduction

"There are only four kinds of people in the world: those who have been caregivers, those who are currently caregivers, those who will be caregivers, and those who will need caregivers."
— First Lady Rosalynn Carter

This book was written specifically to help family caregivers. It has answers to pressing questions about caregiving. Many of you have been thrust into the role of caregiver, prepared or not. Unprepared, your biggest challenge may be trying to figure out what resources are available, how to find them and what do with them.

Caregiving is an important and challenging job. Even though it can be rewarding, it can also be extremely stressful. So, no matter where you are in the process of caregiving, just starting out or in the middle of it, this book will help you meet everyday challenges with confidence and understanding.

The first half of this book offers easy-to-understand answers to the most frequently-asked questions asked by caregivers. The second half of the book contains forms you can use to build your own caregiving organizer. This book provides the tools, information and tips you need to get started with successful caregiving. It offers useful guidance, advice, tips, reassurance and support.

I am always interested in hearing from readers. If you would like to share an experience, offer a suggestion, or pose a question, please write to: EKLEKTIKA Press, Inc., P.O.Box 157, Chelsea, MI 48118. You are invited to click by our web site and join our community to share your caregiving stories and concerns. We want to hear from you.

www.MeAndMyCaregivers.com

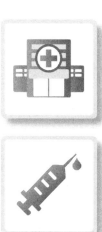
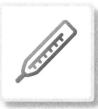
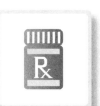
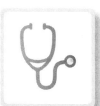
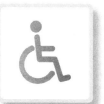

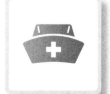

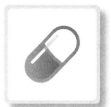
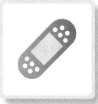
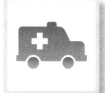

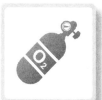
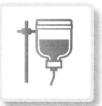

Part 1

Frequently Asked Questions

About Caregivers and Caregiving

The caregiver role is complex and differs for everyone depending on the needs of the care-receiver/patient. Many times, in the beginning, there may only be a few needs, such as providing transportation or helping with shopping or cooking. Over time, needs increase, requiring additional services, until the care-receiver is fully dependent on the caregiver.

Family caregivers are usually related to the care-receiver as spouses, mates, children, in-laws, or other family members. Sometimes, caregivers are not related at all, but assist as good friends or neighbors.

Most caregiving takes place in one of three settings: the care-receiver remains at home, the care-receiver moves in with a friend or family member, or the care-receiver moves into a residential setting.

Caregiving can increase anxiety and distress, particularly when the responsibilities of work, marriage, child rearing are combined with caregiving of an older family member.

1. Who is a caregiver?

A caregiver is a person who takes care of the needs of a child or dependent adult. According to the Family Caregiver Alliance, a caregiver is anyone who provides assistance to someone else that is in some degree incapacitated and needs help. This book's focus is geared toward caregiving of an elder family member.

2. What is the difference between a "formal" and "informal" caregiver?

A paid caregiver is usually referred to as a "formal" caregiver. This person provides non-medical and/or medical care and may be professionally trained and certified. Most unpaid, family caregivers are considered "informal" caregivers.

3. What is a Family Caregiver?

A family caregiver is an adult family member, or another individual, who is an informal provider of in-home and community care to an older individual. This is a broad definition. In addition to close family members, other relatives, friends, neighbors, domestic partners, and others often share the burden of caring for their loved ones.

These individuals may be primary or secondary caregivers, full or part time, and may live with the care-receiver or live separately.

4. How many caregivers are there?

According to the National Family Caregivers Association:

- More than 50 million people provide care for a chronically ill, disabled or aged family member or friend during any given year.
- Approximately 60% of family caregivers are women.
- 30% of family caregivers caring for seniors are themselves aged 65 or over; another 15% are between the ages of 45 to 54.
- 17% of family caregivers are providing 40 hours of care a week or more.
- The value of the services family caregivers provide for "free" is estimated to be $306 billion a year. That is almost twice as much as is actually spent on homecare and nursing home services combined ($158 billion).
- The need for family caregivers will increase in the years ahead. People over 65 are expected to increase at a 2.3% rate, but the number of family members available to care for them will only increase at a 0.8% rate.
- In 2000, 54 million people were involved in some level of caregiving and spent, on average, more than 20 hours per week in this capacity.
- The average American woman can expect to spend more years caring for her parents than she did her children.
- An estimated 21 million Americans provide care to a relative, friend or neighbor who is 50 or older.
- The typical caregiver of an older adult is around 46 years old.
- Men are taking responsibility for the same everyday task as women, including grocery shopping, managing medications and transportation. Women are more involved in personal care such as bathing, dressing, and toileting.

5. Is family caregiving a new phenomenon?

Not really. In years past families have always taken care of their severely ill or disabled, loved ones. Now, family caregiving has become an essential part of our health and long-term care system. Family caregiving has become more than an act of love and family responsibility. It has become a societal issue. Eventually it will affect every American, in one way or another.

We are living much longer. People are living to experience chronic illness. There is a much larger aged population. Hospital stays are shorter. Healthcare costs have skyrocketed. These are just a few of the reasons why there is a greater need for family caregivers today than in years past.

6. Who becomes a caregiver?

People generally become family caregivers as a result of crisis situations, such as when a parent suffers a debilitating illness or accident. More women than men are caregivers, even though the numbers of male caregivers are increasing.

7. What is the National Caregiver Support Act?

The National Family Caregiver Support Program (NFCSP), funded by the Federal Older Americans Act, Title III E, helps persons any age who serve as unpaid caregivers for persons sixty or older. The goal of this program is to relieve the emotional, physical, and financial hardships of providing continual care.

The National Family Caregiver Support Program provides these services:

- Information to caregivers about available services.
- Assistance to caregivers in gaining access to supportive services.
- Individual counseling, organization of support groups, and caregiver training to assist caregivers in making decisions and solving problems relating to their roles.
- Respite care to enable caregivers to be temporarily relieved from their caregiving responsibilities.
- Supplemental services, on a limited basis, to complement the care provided by caregivers.

Your local Area Agency on Aging is one of the first resources a caregiver should contact when help is needed. Almost every state has one or more Area Agency on Aging, which serves local communities, older residents, and their families.

In a few states, the State Unit or Office on Aging serves as the Area Agency on Aging. Local Area Agencies on Aging are generally listed in the city or county government sections of the telephone directory under "Aging" or "Social Services."

8. Do you have to have a certain personality style to be a good caregiver?

Not everyone is suited to caregiving. Take an honest appraisal of your capabilities. What can you handle physically, emotionally, and mentally?

An impulsive choice to be a caregiver can lead to abuse of the care-receiver, nervous breakdowns, poor health, and fiscal fraud.

It is imperative that each caregiver has a good emotional support system.

9. What is the amount and type of care provider by a caregiver?

Role expectations are not always clear. New rules and roles should be defined early on, within the family. This can be a stressful situation, creating conflicts within the caregiver because of personal expectations about appropriate ways to perform as a spouse or adult child. Many times it is difficult to change family roles that were developed over a long period of time.

In many families, there is a lot of friction that increases as changes occur. Many family situations are not warm, loving, open, friendly or cooperative.

While the average caregiver provides care for 18 hours a week, 25 percent of American households spend even more time caregiving. More than four million households provide at least 40 hours per week of unpaid, family assistance to older relatives.

The amount of time spent caregiving increases greatly as cognitive impairment of the care-receiver worsens. Among people over age 70, those with no dementia receive an average of 4.6 hours per week of care, while those with mild dementia receive 13.1 hours of care weekly. For individuals with severe dementia, hours of informal care received rises to almost 46 hours per week.

Transportation, grocery shopping, and household chores are the most common tasks that caregivers perform. A third of the caregivers help with medications, pills, or injections.

Other common tasks involved in caregiving include: personal care such as bathing, dressing, eating, toileting, companionship to support emotional and mental health, and household chores such as cooking and cleaning.

10. What is the average duration of providing caregiving services?

The duration of caregiving can last from less than a year to more than 40 years. In a recent national study, over 40 percent of caregivers had been providing assistance for five or more years, and nearly one-fifth had been doing so for 10+ years.

11. What is the geographic distance between caregiver and care-receiver?

The majority of caregivers live within twenty minutes of the care-receiver. One-quarter of care-receivers live with the caregiver and another one-fifth live within an hour of the care-receiver. The remaining 15 percent of caregivers live more than an hour from the care-receiver.

12. What is considered long-distance caregiving?

Long-distance caregivers are generally defined as living more than one hour from the older adult needing assistance. Estimates of the number of long-distance caregivers in the USA who are caring for an older family member range from five to seven million.

13. Is part of caregiving just a role reversal of parent and child?

No, absolutely not. As the parent's dependence increases, it is natural for adult children to find themselves unable to communicate in familiar ways with their parent. It is important that the child not reverse the roles even though the parent may appear to revert to childlike behaviors. The parent must remain an adult and must be treated accordingly. It is important for the parent to be treated with respect and dignity.

14. What are the top caregiver concerns about becoming a full time caregiver?

The top fears include: worry, fear, embarrassment, shame, grief, anger, depression, helplessness, and guilt.

Caregivers worry that their best efforts may not be enough or good enough. They worry about their care-receiver's fate, as well as, their own fate. They even worry that the care-receiver will die on their watch. They are concerned that other family members and outsiders will fault them for their efforts. The role of caregiver is not always an easy one.

Providing care for someone you love who is no longer able to take care of himself, produces a wide range of emotions. It's natural to feel sadness and grief for your loved one's losses and for the loss of your own previous life. More emotions may surface after you've been a caregiver for an extended period of time or the amount of care increases. You may have days when you feel angry, resentful, impatient, guilty, ashamed, lonely, and even sorry for yourself.

You may find some of your thoughts appalling. Some of these thoughts may seem extremely negative or even abnormal. For example, you may dream about quitting your job, or wishing your patient would die.

These feelings aren't self-centered or mean-spirited. It is a normal response to the extreme changes that providing care brings to your life.

As a caregiver, you give a great deal of your time and energy to someone else's needs, and often ignore your own. When difficult emotions surface, remember that you have your own needs. Let these feelings prompt you to do something for yourself — even if it's only taking 15 minutes to decompress by taking some quiet time or doing something relaxing.

15. Is it normal for caregivers to have both negative and positive feelings about their job?

Yes. It is easy to have and express feelings of love and caring. However, it may not be so easy to admit negative feelings that are less socially acceptable.

16. What are some of the negative feelings often expressed by caregivers?

Because each caregiving situation is different, the following feelings may not be experienced by everyone. It is important that all caregivers have someone they can talk to about their feelings. It is important to vocalize what you are feeling.

Anger: Many caregivers feel trapped. They feel angry that other family members don't contribute in caregiving. They feel angry at the care-receiver's demands and behaviors. They feel anger toward the health-care system and the rest of the care team. They feel angry about the high costs associated with caregiving.

Depression: Because caregiving can be both emotionally and physically draining, it is easy to become depressed. It is easy to feel overwhelmed.

Symptoms of depression may include:

- Sadness
- Loss of interest or pleasure in activities you used to enjoy
- Change in weight
- Difficulty in sleeping or oversleeping
- Energy loss
- Feelings of worthlessness
- Thoughts of death or suicide

Embarrassment: They often feel embarrassed by the care-receiver's behavior, especially with moderate or greater cognitive failure of the care-receiver.

Fear: Family caregivers fear they may be the next family member to need a caregiver. They fear they may not be able to handle the situation. They fear being graded on their "caregiving performance." They fear they will never have a normal life again. They fear the care-receiver will die before other family members can get there.

Guilt: They feel guilty for wanting their role as caregiver to end. They feel guilty for wishing the care-receiver would die. They feel guilty for not being able to do more.

Helplessness: The situation is too great and there is no way to control it.

Shame: Caregivers often feel ashamed of the care-receiver's failings — for what they have become. The caregiver also feels ashamed for having these negative feelings.

Worry: They worry that later they may feel like they didn't do enough.

Grief: Caregivers grieve for the way the care-receiver used to be, for the way things used to be. They grieve for lost relationships. Chronic grief occurs when there is one loss after another, with no time to complete the grieving process in between losses.

17. What is the Caregiver's Bill of Rights?

The Caregiver's Bill of Rights was written by Jo Horne. This is a good reminder that you have rights, too.

Caregiver's Bill of Rights

I have the right:	To take care of myself. This is not an act of selfishness. It will enable me to take better care of my loved one.
I have the right:	To seek help from others even though my loved one may object. I recognize the limits of my own endurance and strength.
I have the right:	To maintain facets of my own life that do not include the person I care for, just as I would if he or she were healthy. I know that I do everything that I reasonably can for this person, and I have the right to do some things for myself.
I have the right:	To get angry, be depressed and express other difficult emotions occasionally.
I have the right:	To reject any attempt by my loved one (either conscious or unconscious) to manipulate me through guilt, anger or depression.
I have the right:	To receive consideration, affection, forgiveness and acceptance from my loved one for as long as I offer these qualities in return.
I have the right:	To take pride in what I am accomplishing and to applaud the courage it sometimes takes to meet the needs of my loved one.
I have the right:	To protect my individuality and my right to make a life for myself that will sustain me when my loved one no longer needs my full-time help.
I have the right:	To expect and demand that as new strides are made in finding resources to aid physically and mentally impaired persons in our country, similar strides will be made toward aiding and supporting caregivers.

About Care-Receivers

More than likely, if we live long enough, we will need the help and assistance of others. Initially it may only be help with housekeeping or transportation tasks. Our daily care and level of needs will change as we age.

18. Who is the typical elderly care-receiver/patient?

Americans who are looked after by others have an average age of 77. Four in ten are older than age 75, and 24 percent are older than age 85.

The vast majority of care-receivers are cared for by a relative; 15 percent by a friend. 31 percent are taken care of by their daughter or son, 9 percent by their daughter-in-law or son-in-law, 12 percent by a grandchild, and 5 percent by a spouse.

Most care-receivers do not live with their caregiver. Only 20 percent do, while 37 percent live with another family member or friend, and 17 percent live alone either in an apartment or a retirement community.

19. Who is being cared for and what are the forecasted future trends?

- Nearly 40 percent of older people living in the community — 12 million people age 65 and older — are limited by chronic conditions. Of these, 3 million (or 10 percent of older people) are unable to perform activities of daily living.
- An estimated 10 percent of people 65 year of age and older, and nearly half of those 85 and older, suffer from Alzheimer's Disease.
- Almost 100 million people in the U.S. have one or more chronic conditions. Over the next twenty-five years this number is expected to increase to 134 million Americans.
- Today there are 35 million people over 65 years of age living in the US. This amount will double to more than 70 million American citizens over 65 years by 2030.
- People are more likely to have older people in their families today than in the past.
- By 2030, when the baby boomers reach age 65, 1 in 5 Americans will be at least 65, for a total of about 70 million older people — more than twice the number in 1996.
- Five social trends may affect the supply of caregivers in the future: 1) increasing divorce and remarriage rates; 2) increasing geographic mobility; 3) decreasing family size; 4) delayed childbearing; and 5) more women in the workplace.
- In the twenty-first century the demands placed on family and other informal caregivers are likely to escalate, affecting nearly every American family.
- With extended life expectancies, baby boomers will create a significant demand for cost-effective alternatives to nursing home care.
- Already, one in three Americans — over 50 million care for a family member or friend. Of those caregivers, 40% are themselves over 55 years of age.
- 54% of people 65+ have at least one disability (physical or non-physical) and 73.6% of 80+ have at least one disability.
- The population aged 85 and older is currently the fastest growing segment of the older adult population in the nation.
- In 2011, the "baby boom" generation will begin to turn 65, and by 2030, it is projected that one in five people will be age 65 or older. The size of the older adult population is projected to double over the next 30 years, growing to 70 million by 2030, twice what it was in 1990.
- Nearly one-quarter (22.9%) of all people 65 and over in this country are functionally disabled or currently in need of some form of long-term care. The best-case scenario projects that by the year 2040 the population of severely disabled elderly (meaning they will need help with personal activities of daily living) will increase by 90%.
- Caregiving for seniors with dementia is less frequent among extended families, likely due to the greater commitment and involvement required in caring for recipients who have psychological illness.

20. What are some characteristics of difficult care-receivers?

It is common for care-receivers to resist what is happening to them. As the person loses control over most parts of daily life, good self-esteem may be replaced with frustration, anger, fear, shame, guilt or embarrassment.

Usually the person becomes more isolated as a result of feelings of helplessness, depression and confusion.

Many times complaining and anger become coping mechanisms. These behaviors can be very taxing to the caregiver.

21. What are the feelings likely to be experienced by care-receivers?

The care-receiver has many of the same feelings as the caregiver.

Anger and Frustration: The care-receiver doesn't like being confined, limited or controlled. He/she doesn't like to be treated as a child.

Embarrassment: Because of the need for personal care, care-receivers often feel embarrassment, coupled with confusion and depression.

Fear: Most people experience some level of fear of what their future may hold. There is also fear associated with loss of control and privacy. The care-receiver feels uncomfortable because his/her familiar role is gone; and his/her power and influence is gone. In general, the loss of independence can generate feelings of fear.

22. Can loss of independence trigger a grieving period?

Yes. All kinds of losses besides death can cause grief reactions. The elements of grief are similar regardless of the type of loss. In fact, grief is very common to the aging person.

Below, is a list of the most commonly experienced phases of grief. Some people take more time than others going through each phase. Grief should never be denied.

- **Shock/denial:** Immediately after learning about a loss, a person tends to be temporarily stunned or disbelieving.
- **Emotional Release:** Next there may be tears, crying, shouting, or venting of the experience of the loss.
- **Depression, Loneliness, Isolation:** A person may experience an "aloneness' with the loss, with no sense of hope for the future.
- **Physical Symptoms:** A person may experience a change in eating and sleeping habits.
- **Panic:** Feelings about the loss disturb the ability to concentrate on anything except the loss.
- **Guilt and Regrets:** A person may feel guilty about everything related to the circumstances of the loss.
- **Hostility, Anger:** This may be a good sign that the grief is being directed outward rather than being contained inside.
- **Discomfort with Normal Activities:** There is a desire to return to normal activities, even though attempts to return are stressful.
- **Hope:** There is a desire for a future and a brief glimpse that better things are possible.
- **Acceptance:** Acceptance comes with the adjustment to reality.
- **Integration:** A person adjusts his life to reality, but the experience has left him different than he was before.

23. Do most care-receivers always become impatient and irritable?

No. Scientists have discovered that an individual's personality and character do not significantly change with the passage of time and remain fairly consistent from adulthood into old age.

However, debilitating illness may strip away the person's finer character attributes. Caregiver's should not expect a grateful response to their caregiving. The truly sensitive caregiver will find a way to nurture the care-receiver's sense of dignity and self worth regardless of the care-receiver's reactions.

> **NOTE:**
>
> Depression is sometimes misdiagnosed as dementia or Alzheimer's, but there are differences. It is important to get a correct diagnosis for any suspected of having depression, dementia or Alzheimer's

Health Issues Associated with Aging

There are changes that occur normally with advancing years. These anticipated changes may require some adjustments in lifestyle, but are not the equivalent of illness. (This is not a comprehensive list.)

24. What are some of the physical changes associated with aging?

General changes: Body composition changes as we age. There is less fluid, more fiber, more fat, a reduced ability to maintain homeostasis, and a decreased intensity of response.

Cardiovascular system: There is longer time needed to return to normal after exercise and blood pressure tends to rise 8-10 points.

Respiratory system: There is decreased lung capacity, less lung flexibility, decreased muscle (chest wall) strength, decreases exhalation, and a less effective cough mechanism.

Urinary system: The kidneys have a decreased capacity to filter waste and medications, blood flow to the kidneys is decreased, and bladder capacity and control is decreased.

Digestive system: Less saliva is produced. There is less gastric acid, and generally slower, less effective digestive processes.

Musculoskeletal system: There is a decrease in muscle strength, loss of bone density, and wear and tear on joints.

Nervous system: There is slower nerve conduction, sleep patterns change, changes in short term memory functions, and changes in speed of response.

Sexuality: There is less intensity of response and less speed of response.

Eyes: There is lower adaptation to changes in light, reduced night vision, increased sensitivity to glare. There are more cases of glaucoma and cataracts.

Ears: The ability to hear high frequencies is diminished or lost altogether.

Taste and Smell: There are fewer taste buds, and decreased sense of smell. These together may decrease pleasure in food.

Touch: There is reduced sensation, particularly in palms of the hands and soles of the feet, and increased difficulty in use of fingers.

25. What are some of the common illnesses and diseases of older people?

These are just a few of the diseases you should be aware.

Alzheimer's Disease: Alzheimer's is a neurological disorder characterized by slow, progressive memory loss due to a gradual loss of brain cells. Alzheimer's disease significantly affects cognitive (thought) capabilities and, eventually, affected individuals become incapacitated.

Anemia: Anemia occurs when there is an insufficient amount of red blood cells in the body. Red blood cells are important to transport oxygen (using hemoglobin) to various parts of your body.

Arthritis: Arthritis is inflammation of a joint, usually accompanied by pain, swelling, and stiffness, and resulting from infection, trauma, degenerative changes, metabolic disturbances, or other causes. It occurs in various forms, such as bacterial arthritis, osteoarthritis, or rheumatoid arthritis.

Atherosclerosis: Atherosclerosis is a process of progressive thickening and hardening of the walls of medium-sized and large arteries as a result of fat deposits on their inner lining.

Bedsores: Bedsores, also called pressure sores, are ulcers (sores) caused by prolonged pressure or rubbing on vulnerable areas of the body.

Cancer: In general, cancer is any malignant growth or tumor caused by abnormal and uncontrolled cell division; it may spread to other parts of the body through the lymphatic system or the blood stream.

Cardiovascular Disease: Cardiovascular Disease is disease affecting the heart or blood vessels. Cardiovascular diseases include arteriosclerosis, coronary artery disease, heart valve disease, arrhythmia, heart failure, hypertension, orthostatic hypotension, shock, endocarditis, diseases of the aorta and its branches, disorders of the peripheral vascular system, and congenital heart disease.

Chronic Obstructive Pulmonary Disease (COPD): Chronic Obstructive Pulmonary Disease is a generic term for lung disease. Two of the most common cases are Chronic Bronchitis and Emphysema.

Congestive Heart Failure: Congestive heart failure (CHF), or heart failure, is caused by loss of pumping power by the heart, resulting in fluids collecting in the body. Congestive heart failure often develops gradually over several years, although it also can happen suddenly.

Constipation: Constipation is a common digestive system problem in which you have infrequent bowel movements, pass hard stools, or strain during bowel movements.

Dehydration: Dehydration means your body does not have as much water and fluids as it should. Dehydration can be caused by losing too much fluid, not drinking enough water or fluids, or both. Vomiting and diarrhea are common causes.

Dementia: Dementia is a word for a group of symptoms caused by disorders that affect the brain. It is not a specific disease. People with dementia may not be able to think well enough to do normal activities, such as getting dressed or eating. They may lose their ability to solve problems or control their emotions. Their personalities may change. They may become agitated or see things that are not there.

Memory loss is a common symptom of dementia. However, memory loss by itself does not mean you have dementia. People with dementia have serious problems with two or more brain functions, such as memory and language.

Depression: Depression is a serious medical illness that involves the brain. It's more than just a feeling of being "down in the dumps" or "blue" for a few days. The feelings do not go away. They persist and interfere with your everyday life. Symptoms can include :

- Sadness
- Loss of interest or pleasure in activities you used to enjoy
- Change in weight
- Difficulty sleeping or oversleeping
- Energy loss
- Feelings of worthlessness
- Thoughts of death or suicide

Diabetes: Diabetes is a disease in which the body does not produce or properly use insulin. Insulin is a hormone that is needed to convert sugar, starches and other food into energy needed for daily life.

Hemorrhoids: Hemorrhoids are inflamed and swollen veins around the lower rectum.

Huntington Disease: Huntington's disease (Huntington's chorea) is a progressive, degenerative disease that causes certain nerve cells in your brain to waste away. As a result, you may experience uncontrolled movements, emotional disturbances and mental deterioration.

Hypertension: High blood pressure or hypertension means high pressure (tension) in the arteries. The arteries are the vessels that carry blood from the pumping heart to all of the tissues and organs of the body

Osteoporosis: Osteoporosis is the thinning of bone tissue and loss of bone density over time.

Parkinson's Disease: Parkinson's disease is a disorder of the brain characterized by shaking (tremor) and difficulty with walking, movement, and coordination. The disease is associated with damage to a part of the brain that is involved with movement.

TIA: A transient ischemic attack is a "mini-stroke" caused by temporary disturbance of blood supply to an area of the brain, which results in a sudden, brief decrease in brain function.

Urinary Tract Infection: A urinary tract infection, or UTI, is an infection that can happen anywhere along the urinary tract -- the kidneys, the ureters (the tubes that take urine from each kidney to the bladder), the bladder, or the urethra (the tube that empties urine from the bladder to the outside).

26. Is confusion a "normal" part of aging?

No, just because you are old doesn't mean you are confused. Confusion can originate from many treatable causes such as infection, poor nutrition, depression, undiagnosed illness, or inappropriate use of medications.

Prevalence of confusion increases with age — 20% of those over 80 show some signs of confusion. Approximately one half of these are related to dementing illnesses such as Alzheimer's Disease.

27. What are some behaviors that may indicate confusion?

Behaviors of the confused may include:

- Cannot answer questions
- Cannot understand complex commands
- Disorientation
- Fails to follow the gist of the conversation
- Loss of power of independent thought
- Loss of reasoning ability

- No recent memory
- Poor attention span
- Poor time sense
- Unreliable memory

28. What can I do to help a confused person?

Without criticism or judgment, accept the impaired person as he/she is now. Attempt to alleviate his/her anxiety. Touch is very helpful. Maintaining a routine or predictable schedule will help to increase a sense of security.

It is important that the care-receiver is provided with adequate stimulation to prevent apathy and withdrawal. Keep the care-receiver busy with activities, visitors, and simple tasks.

The caregiver may need additional help to cope with the daily problems and situations he/she is faced with. Be sure to talk with the care-receiver's doctor about any changes in behavior.

> **Tip:**
>
> **Healthy Aging: Ask the Doctor**
> 1. Exercise
> 2. Dietary Advice
> 3. Nutritional Supplements
> 4. Alcohol Consumption
> 5. Smoking

> **When To See A Doctor**
>
> Consult with a doctor when memory lapses become frequent enough to concern you or the care-receiver — whether the difficulty came on gradually or suddenly.

First Aid/Emergencies/CPR

There are generally two types of first aid, emergency and basic. You will find some of each in this section. **This is not a complete guide to first aid or emergency care.** You should attend both a first aid training course and an artificial resuscitation training course before you start caregiving. The American Red Cross and many hospitals offer these courses.

If an emergency arises and you are unsure of how to handle it, call 911.

29. What is first aid?

First aid is emergency care given immediately to an injured person. The purpose of first aid is to minimize injury and future disability. In serious cases, first aid may be necessary to keep the victim alive.

30. What are the guidelines for giving first aid?

Your first response during the beginning stage of an emergency is critical. Remember this:

A - Ask for help.

I - Intervene.

D - Do no further harm.

Time is important. The more quickly you recognize an emergency and the faster you call for help, the sooner the care-receiver will get help.

31. When should I call for an ambulance?

Call for an ambulance if a person:

- Is unconscious or doesn't wake or respond when shaken.
- Has difficulty breathing, shortness of breath or blue lips or mouth.
- Has chest or upper abdominal pain or pressure or if heart attack is suspected– crushing chest pain that lasts more than five minutes. The pain may spread to arms and jaw.
- Faints.
- Has sudden dizziness, weakness or change in vision.
- Has a change in mental status (such as unusual behavior, confusion, difficulty arousing).
- Has sudden, severe pain anywhere in the body.
- Has bleeding that won't stop.
- Has severe or persistent vomiting.
- Coughs up or vomits blood.
- Has suicidal or homicidal feelings.
- Has burns which are bigger than the size of a hand and/or cause severe pain that is not relieved with simple painkillers, or if the person has difficulty breathing.
- Has choking, especially if the person is unable to talk, cry or breathe.
- Has stroke (possible), especially if the person experiences numbness, loss of function of hand, arm or leg, slurred speech, facial droop or severe abrupt headache.
- Has pain (severe) after a fall or injury, when the person is unable to sit up, stand or walk.
- Drug overdose or poisoning, whether you know for sure or just suspect an overdose.
- Has allergic reaction, especially with difficulty breathing or loss of consciousness.
- Electrical shock of any kind.
- Has trauma (injury), which is severe, especially to the head, neck, chest or abdomen.

32. What if the care-receiver has signed a DNR order?

If the care-receiver has signed a Do Not Resuscitate (DNR) order, have it available to show the paramedics. The order must go with the patient. It is imperative that the DNR order must stay with the patient at all times.

33. What basic first aid should I know how to perform?

First aid begins with action, which in itself has a calming effect. First aid is the assistance given to an injured or sick person in need of urgent medical assistance. It applies to a broad range of medical situations and consists both of specific knowledge and and the ability to assess a situation and make appropriate decisions (such as when to call for emergency medical assistance).

Preparedness is a key element of first aid. You should know how to perform cardiopulmonary resuscitation (CPR). In addition, you should know how to perform the Heimlich Maneuver to assist choking victims.

First aid may be required for medical emergencies such as heart attack, stroke, or seizures as well as for minor medical conditions like nosebleed and mild allergic reactions.

Environmental injuries (sunburn, poison ivy, heat exhaustion, frostbite, bee or insect stings) and traumatic injuries (strains, sprains, burns, puncture wounds, and cuts as well as more severe internal injuries) are other situations where first aid skills can be invaluable.

Especially when caring for the elderly, even a small, seemingly unimportant injury, such as a splinter wound or a puncture wound, can quickly lead to an infection, threatening the health and limb of the patient. Even the smallest scratch is large enough for dangerous germs to enter, and in large bruises or deep cuts, germs come in by the millions. Immediate examination and treatment is necessary for every injury.

Regardless of your level of skill or degree of first aid training, if you find yourself in a true medical emergency, **always call 911 for emergency medical assistance immediately.**

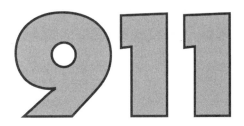

34. What items should be included in the home first aid kit?

- first-aid manual
- your list of emergency phone numbers
- list of current medications
- sterile gauze
- adhesive tape
- adhesive bandages in several sizes
- elastic bandage
- antiseptic wipes/disinfectant for cleaning wounds
- soap
- antibiotic cream (triple-antibiotic ointment)
- antiseptic solution (like hydrogen peroxide)
- hydrocortisone cream (1%)
- acetaminophen and ibuprofen
- extra prescription medications
- tweezers and needle
- sharp scissors
- safety pins
- disposable instant cold packs
- calamine lotion
- alcohol wipes or ethyl alcohol
- thermometer
- eye pads
- plastic/disposable gloves (at least 2 pairs)
- flashlight and extra batteries
- mouthpiece for administering CPR (can be obtained from your local Red Cross)
- blanket (stored nearby)

35. What is Cardiopulmonary Resuscitation (CPR)?

Cardiopulmonary resuscitation (CPR) is a lifesaving technique useful in many emergencies, including heart attack, in which someone's breathing or heartbeat has stopped. CPR involves a combination of mouth-to-mouth rescue breathing and chest compression that keeps oxygenated blood flowing to the brain and other vital organs until other medical treatment can restore a normal heart rhythm.

When the heart stops, the absence of oxygenated blood can cause irreparable brain damage in only a few minutes. Death will occur within eight to 10 minutes. Time is critical when you're helping an unconscious person who isn't breathing.

To learn CPR properly, take an accredited first-aid training course, including CPR and how to use an automated external defibrillator (AED).

36. What is the Heimlich Maneuver?

The Heimlich Maneuver is a series of under-the-diaphragm abdominal thrusts. It's recommended for helping a person who's choking on a foreign object (foreign-body airway obstruction).

The Heimlich Maneuver lifts the diaphragm and forces enough air from the lungs to create an artificial cough. The cough is intended to move and expel an obstructing foreign body in an airway. Each thrust should be given with the intent of removing the obstruction.

> **For more information on the Heimlich Maneuver:**
> - Check with your local Red Cross
> - Ask your doctor
> - Check for classes at your local hospital or fire department
> - Check online

37. How are seniors most likely to need first aid?

For seniors, falls in and around the home are the most frequently occurring accident. Here are some tips to help prevent falls:

- Have the care-receiver's hearing and eyesight tested. Inner ear problems can affect balance. Vision problems make it difficult to see potential hazards.
- Watch alcohol intake, especially if the care-receiver is on any medications.
- Exercise regularly (with the doctor's permission) to improve muscle flexibility and strength.
- Have a lamp or light switch near the care-receiver's bed that he/she can reach without getting out of bed.
- Keep flashlights handy in each room.
- Use night lights in every room.
- Add grab bars in shower, tub and toilet areas.
- Use bath mats with suction cups.
- Keep telephone and electrical cords out of pathways.
- Have care-receiver use adaptive devices to help with balance: cane, walker, wheelchair.

38. What is the File of Life™?

The File of Life card enables medics to obtain a quick medical history when the patient is unable to offer one. The card, which is kept in a red plastic pocket labeled FILE OF LIFE, lists the patient's name, emergency medical contacts, insurance policy and social security number, health problems, medications, dosages, allergies, recent surgeries, religion, doctor's name and health care proxy. The entire pocket is held, with a magnet to the outside of the refrigerator.

Emergency personnel have been trained to check the patient's refrigerator for this information.

A File of Life magnet can be purchased from www.MeAndMyCaregivers.com. For more information about this program, visit: www.folife.org.

> **TIP:**
>
> Post emergency numbers — for fire, police, ambulance, and poison control — in large red writing near all phones.

Getting Ready

Becoming a caregiver is a big undertaking and it doesn't come with a specific job description. Often the role of caregiving is unexpected and comes at a time when you are unprepared. Keep in mind, that even the most prepared caregivers face new challenges everyday.

This part of the book is designed to help you "get ready" to move into the caregiver role.

Communication and Decision Making

Gaining the cooperation and help of family members can make your caregiving job easier. Being able to articulate your feelings and needs will make your job easier, too.

39. How do I become a good communicator?

Being a good communicator and decision maker will help you to be a better caregiver. Keep in mind that you may have to develop a new style of communication in order to draw family members together for decision making. There are a number of reasons why family members may have difficulty with communication.

Communication is the exchange of thoughts, messages, or information, as by speech, signals, writing or behavior; interpersonal rapport. Communication within families is special and unique. Over the years family members develop their own style of communicating. Sometimes a facial expression or gesture is worth a thousand words.

This style will either be a strength or weakness, at a time when the family needs to come together and make decisions about an aging family member. Many family members find that their personal communication style has changed over the years, others find that their poor communication style has intensified.

It is important to be sensitive to the needs of others. Good communication requires both good speaking and good listening skills. Because decision making in stressful situations tends to be difficult, it is important to employ good communication techniques.

40. What can I do to encourage better communication between family members?

Families are able to adjust to difficult times in direct proportion to their ability to communicate with each other. Family members can benefit greatly when they can rely on each other as sounding boards to clarify thoughts and plans. Unfortunately, many families have a difficult time communicating with each other.

Be aware that as family members become caught up in their own lives, it is easy to fall into a rut and take each other for granted. Be aware that words, phrases, and even facial expressions that had a shared meaning in the past may have different meanings, now, years later. Be aware that contrary to what we might all wish, magical transformations of family dynamics do not necessarily change as the parent ages. Poor family communication in the past is likely to continue.

The best way to encourage better communication between family members is to be more sensitive to the needs of others and their desire to be understood. You have to be a good listener as well as a good speaker.

Even when families devote time and energy to improving their communication skills, some conflict and misunderstanding should be expected. These situations are a part of almost every family. If there are serious family problems and misunderstandings, it is a good idea to call a family meeting. It may even help to have a neutral mediator present. Give each family member a chance to state their views. Sometimes this is enough to reduce random complaining so important decisions can be made.

41. How can I become a better speaker?

Write your thoughts down on a note card and refer to it when trying to articulate your thoughts. Carefully choose your time and place to have a conversation. When and where can you expect the full attention of the other person? Some things are better said in person rather than over the telephone or through e-mail.

The way we stand, sit or greet another person conveys subtle messages about our expectations and attitudes. Ideally, our stance should convey assertive self-confidence and self-control and not passive or aggressive signals. Check these aspects of your interactions with family members. What impression might they make?

You can improve your chances of being heard if you use "I" statements rather than "you" statements which may be interpreted as blaming statements.

42. How can I be a better listener?

If you are preoccupied it is often better to re-schedule the discussion. To be a better listener, practice these listening keys:

- Listen attentively — just listen.
- Listen actively — pay attention.
- Listen reflectively — be able to paraphrase and say back what the speaker just said.
- Listen slowly.
- Listen deeply — listen well, be able to connect the dots between past, present and future.
- Listen connectively — make meaningful connections.
- Listen openly.
- Listen respectfully — be tolerant even when you don't agree.
- Listen appreciatively — show positive regard.
- Listen intuitively — use your sixth sense to hear underlying messages.

43. Is it important to have a family meeting to establish a strategy for caregiving?

Yes. Meetings may occur occasionally or regularly, be formal or informal. They can be in person, over the phone, on a conference call, or a combination.

Decisions that affect important aspects of someone else's life may be extremely difficult and shouldn't be taken lightly.

Remember, shared decisions generally produce the best results. All participants will feel as if they own the outcome.

44. What are the steps for holding a family meeting or formal decision making process?

Step 1 — Set-up the ground rules. For example, no sidebars, no interruptions, only one person has the floor at a time, etc. Elect one person to lead the meeting and keep everyone on track.

Step 2 — State the situation and select the problem. A good way to begin is by describing the situation. Ask each family member to state the problem as he sees it. You may be surprised to find out the situation seems quite different to each person.

Step 3 — Next, state a goal. What would you like to achieve? It is important to be as specific as possible. In what direction do the caregiver and/or family member want to move? The person's whose life will be most affected by the decision should have a major input regarding the goal, if possible.

Step 4 — Make assessments. Once you have set a goal you may find you need more information. You may need to obtain medical information about the care-receiver. You may need a psychological assessment of the care-receiver. You may need to know financial information about the care-receiver. A social assessment may bring to light additional sources of support and help.

Step 5 — Make an action plan. Once resources and limitations have been assessed, look for other choices that might improve the situation. Your objective is to identify the choice that will have the fewest undesirable consequences and yet be acceptable to as many as possible, and particularly the care-receiver.

Keep in mind, your decision making process may lead to a decision not to act or not to change things.

Step 6 — (Don't skip this step.) Trial period. For a specific length of time, agree to work toward making the Action Plan a success. During this period of time, put aside conflicting ideas.

Step 7 — Evaluation. The final step of decision making is to evaluate the results. One of the major benefits of a trial period and evaluation, is it often redefines the problem. With new information you may have to work through the decision making process again.

45. What are five common roadblocks to family meetings?

1. Family members say things they don't mean.
2. Family members keep secrets. They are afraid to speak out for fear of being blamed or judged.
3. Family members often hide their feelings.
4. Family members make commitments they do not intend to keep or may not be able to keep.
5. Family members make hasty decisions that do not honor the wishes of the care-receiver.

46. What do I do if there is an impasse at the family meeting?

Take a short break. Encourage everyone to keep their hearts open to the process. Don't let fear rule your decisions. Bring in an outside facilitator if necessary.

Assembling the Care Team

Look beyond your family members for help. You will need to enlist the help of others, including professionals.

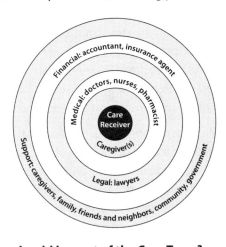

47. Who should be part of the Care Team?

Both the care-receiver and caregiver are important members of the Care Team. However, you can't do this job without the help of others. Others on the team should include doctors and nurses for health management, advisors for financial and tax planning, as well for end-of-life planning. Encourage other family members and/or other caregivers to be a part of the team.

Open communication between team members will help to ensure that the care-receiver gets the best of care. It is important to keep everyone informed of the care-receiver's condition.

Be sure to let family and friends know when you need help. You may need the help of home health aides, housekeeping/chore services, care managers, financial advisors, insurance managers, neighbors, church volunteers, senior centers, transportation services, home maintenance and repair services, personal emergency response systems, hospice care, adult day care or night care programs, or delivered meals.

48. Medical Considerations

Learn as much as you can about the care-receiver's illness and treatment. Information can help you understand what is going on and it can also make talking with the doctor easier.

Make sure you have written permission from the care-receiver to receive medical information. There is a Release of Information Form on page 112. Use it to make more copies. or, you can go to www.MeAndMyCaregivers.com and download additional copies.

49. What is HIPAA?

HIPAA is an acronym for the Health Insurance Portability & Accountability Act of 1996. This Act was introduced in 1996, but not fully implemented until 2003. HIPAA was created to insure that people between jobs would still have access to quality health care coverage, since in the past it was difficult to change insurance carriers without facing lowered coverage or ultra-high premiums. HIPAA was also intended to protect private health care information and create a uniform standard for dispersing personal information.

What does portability mean? Before HIPAA, if a person lost his job and therefore his insurance coverage, the next insurance company he used could classify his health needs as "pre-existing conditions." Doing so allowed the insurance provider to pay little or nothing for services needed to remedy such conditions, despite the fact that the client was paying for the insurance.

By disallowing pre-existing condition policies, requiring new companies to renew insurance policies, and barring carriers from charging higher premiums based on health information, HIPAA plans to make insurance coverage "portable" between companies. This measure is intended to keep people who change jobs from being forced to forgo health insurance due to difficulty in securing coverage or due to insurmountable expense.

What does accountability mean? In regard to HIPAA, accountability refers to the standards by which private health care information is exchanged between insurance companies, health care providers, pharmacies, employers and patients. In the age of technology, electronic transfer of information makes it very easy to violate a patient's privacy, even inadvertently.

HIPAA gives the Department of Health and Human Services the authority to create uniform controls for the management and transfer of sensitive information, including the ability to determine which codes must be used to identify medical and administrative expenses. HIPAA also gives HHS the ability to create a national ID system for clients, health care providers and insurance carriers. Finally, HIPAA gives HHS the power to implement procedures necessary to secure personal information and protect the privacy of health care information.

If you've visited the doctor or a pharmacy, you've probably been asked to sign a form stating that you received this information. Such forms may provide space for you to indicate who may and may not review your personal health care information. While many people simply sign the form, it is a good idea to read the information carefully first. You might be surprised by how and with whom your private health care information is shared!

50. How can I keep up with the care-receiver's medical care?

Start by learning as much as you can about their health, illnesses and treatments. This information will be essential as you help the care-receiver cope with day-to-day concerns, make decisions, and plan for the future.

Record this information in the Family Caregiver Organizer: A Personal and Medical Journal for the Care-receiver and their Caregiver(s) or go to www.MeAndMyCaregivers.com and subscribe to the electronic version and store the records online.

Go along on the care-receiver's doctor's appointments. Keep in mind that you must have permission to have any conversation with the care-receiver's doctor. You will be asked to complete a release form that allows the doctor to discuss his health care with you. Keep the release up-to-date. Ask for a copy to keep in the care-receiver's home records.

51. How can I make the most of a visit with the care-receiver's doctor?

How well you (care-receiver and caregiver) and your doctor talk to each other is one of the most important parts of getting good health care. It takes time and effort on your part, as well as the doctor's.

If you go with the care-receiver to see the doctor, try these tips:

- Before the appointment, ask the care-receiver and other caregivers, if they have any questions or concerns they would like you to bring up. Write them down. Bring a prioritized list of questions and take notes on what the doctor says.
- Bring a copy of the Family Caregiver Organizer to the appointment. If you are not using the journal, make a list of ALL medications the care-receiver is taking, both prescription and over-the-counter, and include dosage and schedule. Don't forget to include medications that may be prescribed by a different doctor.*
- When the doctor asks a question, do not answer for the care-receiver, unless you have been asked to do so.
- Respect the care-receiver's privacy, and leave the room when necessary.

*If you subscribe to the online version of the *Family Caregiver Organizer*, bring the login information with you so the doctor can review the records. (For subscription information, visit www.MeAndMyCaregivers.com).

Legal Issues/End-of-Life Planning

There are several legal issues that are important to every family caring for an elder or impaired member. Even though the laws and legal terminology may vary from state to state, the issues remain the same.

It is important that everyone have an up-to-date will, power of attorney, and advance directives. "Advance Directive" is the generic name for a document that expresses an individual's preferences regarding the acceptance or rejection of medical treatment under certain medical conditions in the event that he/she subsequently becomes unable to make decisions or express his/her wishes.

There are many attorneys who specialize in Elder Law. It is important to learn about the options for end-of-life care, and equally important to comprehend the recommendations that the Care Team provides.

Wills and Trusts

52. What is a will?

A will is a legal document that outlines your wishes for the disposition of your estate after your death.

Here are some basic elements generally included in a will:

- Your name and place of residence.
- A brief description of your assets.
- Names of spouse, children and other beneficiaries such as charities or friends.
- Alternate beneficiaries, in the event, a beneficiary dies before you do.
- Specific gifts, such as an automobile or residence.
- Establishment of trusts, if desired.
- Cancellation of debts owed to you, if desired.
- Name of a personal representative (executor) to manage the state and an alternate if the first is unable or unwilling to serve.
- Name of a guardian for minor children.
- Name of an alternate guardian, in the event your first

choice is unable or unwilling to act.
- Your signature.
- Witnesses' signatures.

53. Do you really need a will?

Other than a properly set up living trust, there is no way for anyone to carry out your intended wishes for disposition of your possessions, without a will.

54. What is an ethical will?

In the law, an ethical will is distinct from its legal counterpart in that it is focused on conveying the writers' values and principals to the next generation. Many ethical wills are written as last letters to loved ones before going into battle or prior to particularly risky surgeries.

55. What is probate?

When a person dies, the legal title of property from their estate has to be transferred to the intended beneficiary via a will. If there is no will, then it is left to the state to determine who is the legal heir to the estate and the property. Collectively, these processes are known as probate.

Probate is a process that is designed to enable the proper transfer of the decedent's estate to the rightful beneficiaries. This process is also used to collect any taxes due on the transfer of the property. Outstanding debts can also be settled through probate, and usually a date is set by which time creditors must file any claims that they have. The balance of the estate or property following settlement of these debts and taxes is then distributed to the beneficiaries. The nature of probate means that if there is no estate or property to be distributed then there is no need to go through probate.

Probate is necessary not only to facilitate distribution of property from the will (if there is a will), but also to allow objections to the will by other parties.

The public are allowed access to probate records, and it therefore possible to see how much estate was left by a deceased individual.

56. What is a trust?

In simple terms, a trust is a relationship in which a person, called a trustor, transfers something of value, called an asset, to another person, called a trustee. The trustee then manages and controls this asset for the benefit of a third person, called a beneficiary. An asset is any kind of property.

57. What is the difference between a trust and a will?

The main difference between a trust and a will is the fact that with a trust, your property won't go through probate when you die. With a will the transfer of property takes place at your death and will need to go through the court system, (probate) to determine the legalities of the will and the properties being dispersed.

When you create a trust you transfer your properties to it while you are still alive and it continues on through your death.

When you create a trust you transfer all your property, assets, bank accounts, securities, real estate to a person or persons you "trust". You no longer own these assets, the "trust" does.

You still have access to all these assets while you are alive. You instruct your Trust to pay out all income to you during your lifetime, and on your death whatever is left would be given to your beneficiaries. You can put instructions in the Trust as to who has access to it. Your property will avoid probate after you die. You will need to appoint a trustee to take care of the Trust and follow its directions. You can be your own trustee. You can be the person that is responsible for taking care of all of the assets while you are alive. You can still control your assets and decide what you want to do with them. After your death your trust would be passed on to a successor trustee that was named in your original trust.

There are many differences with the wording of Trusts and many different types of trusts. However, there are two basic distinctions the Living Trust and the Testamentary Trust. A Living Trust is created and instated while you are alive. A Testamentary Trust is carried out after your death from instructions given while you were alive. There is also the distinction of revocable and irrevocable trusts. A revocable trust can be changed, added to, taken from or stopped at anytime by the person instating it. If the trust does not specifically state that the trust can be revoked or amended, then it is an irrevocable trust and can not be altered, ever.

58. What is the definition of a Conservator?

A Conservator is an individual who has obtained legal authority to manage the estate and financial affairs of an Incapacitated Adult.

59. What is the definition of a Guardian?

A Guardian is an individual who is appointed by the Court to be responsible for the personal affairs of an Incapacitated Adult, including responsibility for making decisions regarding the person's support, care, health, safety, habilitation, education, therapeutic treatment, and if not inconsistent with an order of commitment, regarding the person's residence.

60. What is the difference between a Guardian and a Conservator?

There are several differences between a Guardian and a Conservator; however the primary difference is that a Conservator is responsible for the financial affairs of an Incapacitated Adult whereas the Guardian is only responsible for the personal affairs of an Incapacitated Adult. Additionally, both a Guardian and a Conservator are required to file certain annual reports, however to different entities.

61. What is a Durable Power of Attorney?

A power of attorney is a legal instrument by which a competent person can assign rights for his/her decision making to another adult. The general power of attorney gives a designated person the right to make decisions for the grantor. The person who assigns this power to another must be competent and able to personally exercise responsibility for the delegated decision making.

A durable power of attorney is an instrument that must be executed while an individual is competent, but the rights that it infers to another individual take effect, or remain in effect, even after a disabling condition occurs.

A durable power of attorney provides protection, without court involvement, for the elderly person in the event of limitation of competence at a later date.

62. What is the difference between Power of Attorney and Durable Power of Attorney?

A power of attorney is a legal document that authorizes someone to act for you. You name someone known as an agent or attorney-in-fact (though the person need not be an attorney) who steps into your shoes, legally speaking. You can authorize your agent to do such things as sign checks and tax returns, enter into contracts, buy or sell real estate, deposit or withdraw funds, run a business, or anything else you do for yourself.

A power of attorney can be broad or limited. Since the power-of-attorney document is tailored for its specific purpose, your agent cannot act outside the scope designated in the document. For example, you may own a home in another state that you want to sell. Instead of traveling to that state to complete all the necessary paperwork, you can authorize someone already in that state to do this for you. When the transactions to sell the home are complete, the agency relationship ends, and the agent no longer holds any power.

A regular power of attorney ends when its purpose is fulfilled; or at your incapacity or death.

A durable power of attorney serves the same function as a power of attorney. However, as its name implies, the agency relationship remains effective even if you become incapacitated. This makes the durable power of attorney an important estate planning tool. If incapacity should strike you, your agent can maintain your financial affairs until you are again able to do so, without any need for court involvement. That way, your family's needs continue to be provided for, and the risk of financial loss is reduced. A durable power of attorney ends at your death.

63. What is an Advance Directive?

It is a legal document that tells doctors and health care providers how you want them to carry out medical decisions you have made for future crisis care, if you cannot communicate these decisions for yourself. An Advance Directive is:

- An instruction such as a Durable Power of Attorney for Health Care (DPAHC).
- A directive in accordance with patient self-determination initiatives.
- A living will.
- An oral directive which states either a person's choices for medical treatment, or in the event a person is unable to make treatment choices, designates who will make those decisions.

Under the law in most states, Advance Directives are documents signed by a competent person, over age 18, giving direction to health care providers about treatment choices in certain circumstances. If a person becomes incapacitated and is no longer capable of making his or her own decisions then an Advance Directive maybe used.

A good Advance Directive describes the kind of treatment you would want depending on how sick you are and unlikely to recover, or if you are permanently unconscious. Advance Directives usually tell your doctor that you don't want certain kinds of treatment. However, they can also say that you want a certain treatment no matter how ill you are.

There are two basic types of Advance Directives: a Durable Power of Attorney for Health Care (DPAHC) and a Living Will.

64. What is a Living Will?

A Living Will is the most common type of Advance Directive. It outlines your wishes in writing and tells your doctor or health care provider, your wishes concerning end-of-life medical care. A Living Will pertains to artificial life support and is not implemented until a physician decides that the individual is terminal.

Basically, a Living Will is a document that allows you to decide whether or not to be kept on artificial life support. It can also include your decisions about organ donation or your wishes to die at home rather than in a hospital.

Remember, with a Living Will, you have to make all of these decisions while you are healthy and mentally competent to avoid any confusion about true intent.

65. What are the limitations of Living Wills?

Living Wills are limited in the range of treatment decisions they permit. Living Wills do not apply in emergency situations.

For example, many serious events, such as strokes, Alzheimer's Disease or comas, are not considered terminal diseases by many doctors and, therefore, may not be covered by Living Wills. Or, if you are seriously injured in a car accident, emergency personnel can do everything in their power to save your life.

You should also be aware that each state has different laws concerning Living Wills. Laws in some states are stricter than in others about when a Living Will can be used.

Because of the limited applicability of Living Wills, you are encouraged to also have a Durable Power of Attorney for Health care (DPAHC).

66. What if you do not make a Living Will and become terminally ill and unable to make decisions?

If you have no Living Will in this situation, your treatment decisions will be made, in front of a witness, by the attending doctors and any of the following persons, in the following order:

1. The person you designated in a Power of Attorney, if any.
2. Your court appointed guardian, if any. Your guardian must obtain court approval before making any decisions.
3. Your spouse.
4. Your adult child. However, if you have more than one child, then the decision is to be made by a majority of your available adult children.
5. Your parent or parents.
6. An adult sibling.

67. What is a Durable Power of Attorney for Health Care (DPAHC)?

A Durable Power of Attorney for Health Care may also be referred to as a Health Care (Medical) Power of Attorney.

It is a legal document that you can use to give someone permission to make medical decisions for you if you are unable to make those decisions yourself, temporarily or permanently. The person you name to represent you may be called an agent, health care proxy, patient advocate, or something similar, depending on where you live.

Unlike a Living Will, a DPAHC empowers someone to act as that person's agent.

A DPAHC can be part of another Advance Directive or Living Will, or may be a separate document.

A DPAHC includes situations where you cannot make treatment decisions for yourself, but do not have a terminal condition.

68. Where can I find Advance Directive forms and instructions?

You can get Advance Directive forms from:

- A local hospital.
- Your attorney.
- Long-Term Care Ombudsman program.
- Senior legal service or senior information and referral program, or a local/state medical society.

- Your physician will usually have forms appropriate for your state.
- Some medical centers offer classes in preparing Advance Directives.
- You can get state-specific directives from a lawyer or the public library.

69. What is the difference between a medical proxy and a health care agent?

A health care agent is someone the individual has selected.

A medical proxy is chosen for a person by agreement of the family, or close friend. A medical proxy should be someone who has a close relationship with the patient and who knows that person's medical wishes.

If family and friends cannot decide who a medical proxy should be or, if they disagree with a proxy's decision, they can object and petition the court to request guardianship.

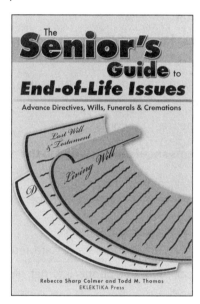

For a more in-depth look at legal issues, take a look at *The Senior's Guide to End-of-Life Issues*.

70. What is a CPR directive?

CPR directives allow people to signal their refusal of cardiopulmonary resuscitation. There are two types of CPR directives:

1. Do Not Resuscitate (DNR): A patient in a hospital or nursing home may have a DNR order that limits the use of resuscitative measures if heartbeat or breathing stops. This should be communicated to the physician in a Durable Power of Attorney for Health Care.

2. Out-of-hospital CPR directive: Some states have statutes that allow an out-of-hospital CPR directive. This type of directive is used by a person who is in the terminal stages of an advanced illness who wants to ensure resuscitative measures are not used by paramedics or other rescue personnel.

In a hospital, DNR orders are part of your medical records and all medical professionals should be aware of them. For out-of-hospital occurrences, say in the home, a proscribed placard may need to be displayed, to ensure your wishes are adhered to. Check your state regulations. In an emergency situation, EMS staff members may not have time to look for, or to evaluate different types of documentation. There is a possibility they may not acknowledge your directive, unless it is in plain sight.

Financial Considerations

When it comes to finances, the typical family caregiver helps with or arranges bill paying, deposits, insurance and benefit claims, savings and investment decisions, housing and adult day-care, tax preparation and many other financial duties.

It is important to plan beyond the completion of legal and medical documents.

To begin:

Gather important financial documents concerning investments (deeds, titles, stocks, bonds, etc.), benefits (pension, IRA accounts, insurance, Social Security, etc.), and expenses (bank accounts, monthly and other bills, etc.), as well as legal documents such as wills or durable powers of attorney.

Consider the costs that will be involved in caring for your loved one, which may include managing their bills, taxes, investments, and benefits. Common expenses that should be taken into consideration when planning include medical costs related to their conditions that exist or may arise, medications, caregiving supplies, care or residential services. Also, especially if your loved one lives with you, consider what costs you yourself have to balance.

Talk with a financial advisor about how you can best put finances in order. An advisor can also help point out if you are eligible for any of the tax deductions that are commonly used by other caregivers.

Other financial considerations:

- Caregivers mean well but often become overly protective and begin making decisions that the care-receiver is fully capable of. The care-receiver, even if physically frail, should always be making his or her own financial decisions. Important decisions should be in consultation with other family members, if appropriate. The caregiver may have to step in if confusion, dementia or mental illness becomes an issue."

- Consider automatic payment of important, recurring bills. You can arrange for water, electric and other utility bills, along with health insurance, mortgage and other regular commitments, to be paid electronically out of your loved one's checking account. This makes bill paying easier and prevents hassles and interruptions in service if required payments aren't made. You also may be able to arrange to be notified if your relative misses a payment.

- Consider the direct deposit of pay and benefit checks into bank and brokerage accounts. Most experts believe direct deposit is safer and more convenient than paper checks. There are no delays in getting funds deposited, no checks are lost in the mail or forgotten at home, and notices about each payment and deposit can be obtained.

- If you must assume full responsibility for a relative's finances, it is recommended that you continue to share information with other family members. Open, honest communication of specific financial decisions as they are made may reduce the possibility of later recriminations.

- You might even want to consider family meetings to discuss finances, just to keep everyone current on spending and income. It's generally also wise to keep good notes about significant discussions you have with family members and the actions taken as a result.

- Think about sharing duties with family and friends. Some regular responsibilities, such as bill paying or deposit making, might be done most efficiently by one person. But don't be shy about asking family, neighbors and old friends to help out where appropriate, from occasional banking matters to basic errands, phone calls and letters. If help is available on a regular basis, that's even better. You'll need a break periodically.

- Be aware of your potential liability. A caregiver may become a joint owner of a checking or savings account, serve as a legal representative (through a power of attorney) or become someone's trustee or guardian. Any time you agree to share responsibility with or for someone else you may be taking on unexpected risks and liabilities. Be prepared for out-of-pocket expenses. Family caregivers don't get paid, often don't get thanked, and frequently don't get reimbursed for long-distance phone calls, travel, groceries, medications, personal care items or other purchases.

71. Is it helpful to perform an estate inventory?

Yes. This information can be helpful to other members of the Care Team.

The following is recommended:

- List of all family members complete with full names and addresses.
- List of prior marriages, noting children from each marriage.
- List of bank accounts and insurance policies, complete with numbers.
- List of all assets, business interests, and credit cards with numbers.
- Identify the location of any safe deposit boxes and keys.
- List any information pertinent to weekly, monthly, or fiscal actions.
- List of computer passwords.

72. What items should be included in the monthly budget?

The following are general categories to be considered:

- Mortgage or rent
- Taxes-property and income-local, state, federal
- Utilities-heat, AC, water, phone, Internet, electricity, TV
- Food-groceries, dining out
- Clothing
- Medications
- Other medical-vision, hearing aids, dental
- Insurance premiums-homeowners, health, car, disability, flood, life, long term care
- Home and yard maintenance
- Home care-caregiving, companions, aides
- Interest payments-credit cards, loans
- Hobbies and pastimes-subscriptions, club dues, classes, gym memberships, equipment
- Pet care

- Entertainment
- Gifts
- Donations
- Other

73. What tax situations should I be aware of?

Consult an Elder Law attorney, accountant or tax professional.

74. How do I avoid a financial crisis?

Advance planning is the best way to avoid a financial crisis. It is important to familiarize yourself with the different options available to you. It is a good idea to have an attorney or accountant review your financial plan. Also, you can contact your local Area Agency on Aging to find out what resources are available to you.

75. What is Medicare?

Medicare is the federal government program that gives you health care coverage if you are 65 or older, or have a disability, no matter what your income. Medicare is divided into three parts: Part A, Part B and Part D.

Medicare Part A covers inpatient hospital, skilled nursing facility, home health and hospice care.

Medicare Part B covers almost all reasonable and necessary medical services, including doctors' services, laboratory and x-ray services, durable medical equipment (wheelchairs, hospital beds), ambulance services, outpatient hospital care, home health care, blood and medical supplies.

Medicare Part D is the new outpatient prescription drug benefit, which is only available through Medicare private drug plans or Medicare private health plans.

(Note: Medicare Part C allows people to get their Medicare-covered services from Medicare private health plans, such as HMOs and PPOs.)

76. Who can get Medicare?

To get more information about medicare, call 1-800-MEDICARE (1-800-633-4227). The helpline has a speech automated system to make it easier for you to get the information you need 24 hours a day, including weekends.

Medicare covers certain medical services and items in hospitals and other settings. Some are covered under Medicare Part A, and some are covered under Medicare Part B. As long as you have both Part A and Part B, these services and items are covered whether you have the Original Medicare Plan, or you belong to a Medicare Advantage Plan (like an HMO or PPO).

Hospital insurance (Part A)

Part A helps cover your inpatient care in hospitals. This includes critical access hospitals and skilled nursing facilities (not custodial or long-term care). It also helps cover hospice care and home health care. You must meet certain conditions to get these benefits.

If you aren't sure if you have Part A, look on your red, white, and blue Medicare card. If you have Part A, "HOSPITAL (PART A)" is printed on your card.

Most people automatically get Part A coverage without having to pay a monthly payment, called a premium. This is because they or a spouse paid Medicare taxes while working.

Most people age 65 or older who are citizens or permanent residents of the United States are eligible for free Medicare hospital insurance (Part A). You are eligible at age 65 if:

- You receive or are eligible to receive Social Security benefits; or
- You receive or are eligible to receive railroad retirement benefits; or
- You or your spouse (living or deceased, including divorced spouses) worked long enough in a government job where Medicare taxes were paid; or
- You are the dependent parent of someone who worked long enough in a government job where Medicare taxes were paid.

If you do not meet these requirements, you may be able to get Medicare hospital insurance by paying a monthly premium. Usually, you can sign up for this hospital insurance only during designated enrollment periods.

NOTE: Even though the full retirement age is no longer 65, you should sign up for Medicare three months before your 65th birthday.

Before age 65, you are eligible for free Medicare hospital insurance if:

- You have been entitled to Social Security disability benefits for 24 months; or
- You receive a disability pension from the railroad retirement board and meet certain conditions; or

- You have Lou Gehrig's disease (amyotrophic lateral sclerosis); or
- You worked long enough in a government job where Medicare taxes were paid and you meet the requirements of the Social Security disability program; or
- You are the child or widow(er) age 50 or older, including a divorced widow(er) of someone who has worked long enough in a government job where Medicare taxes were paid and you meet the requirements of the Social Security disability program.
- You have permanent kidney failure and you receive maintenance dialysis or a kidney transplant and:
  - You are eligible for or receive monthly benefits under Social Security or the railroad retirement system; or
  - You have worked long enough in a Medicare-covered government job; or
  - You are the child or spouse (including a divorced spouse) of a worker (living or deceased) who has worked long enough under Social Security or in a Medicare-covered government job.

Medicare Part A helps to cover your medically necessary:

Blood: Pints of blood you get at a hospital or skilled nursing facility during a covered stay.

Home Health Services: Limited to reasonable and necessary part-time or intermittent skilled nursing care and home health aide services, and physical therapy, occupational therapy, and speech-language pathology ordered by your doctor and provided by a Medicare-certified home health agency. Also includes medical social services, durable medical equipment (such as wheelchairs, hospital beds, oxygen, and walkers), and medical supplies for use at home.

Hospice Care: For people with a terminal illness (less than six months to live). Includes drugs for symptom control and pain relief, medical and support services from a Medicare-approved hospice, and other services not otherwise covered by Medicare (like grief counseling). Hospice care is usually given in your home (may include a nursing facility if this is your home). However, Medicare covers some short-term hospital and inpatient respite care (care given to a hospice patient so that the usual caregiver can rest).

Hospital Stays: Semiprivate room, meals, general nursing, and other hospital services and supplies. This includes inpatient care you get in critical access hospitals and mental health care. This doesn't include private-duty nursing or a television or telephone in your room. It also doesn't include a private room, unless medically necessary. Inpatient mental health care in a psychiatric hospital is limited to 190 days in a lifetime.

Skilled Nursing Facility Care: Semiprivate room, meals, skilled nursing and rehabilitative services, and other services and supplies (only after a three-day inpatient hospital stay for a related illness or injury) for up to 100 days in a benefit period. Note: Medicare doesn't cover long-term care.

Medical insurance (Part B)

Part B helps cover medical services like doctors' services, outpatient care, and other medical services that Part A doesn't cover. Part B is optional. Part B helps pay for medical services and items when they are medically necessary. Part B also covers some preventative services.

You pay the Part B premium each month. In some cases, this amount may be higher if you didn't sign up for Part B when you first became eligible.

You also pay a Part B deductible each year before Medicare starts to pay its share. You may be able to get help from your state to pay this premium and deductible.

If you don't take Part B when you are first eligible, the cost of Part B will go up 10% for each full 12-month period that you could have had Part B but didn't sign up for it, except in special cases. You may have to pay this penalty as long as you have Part B.

Anyone who is eligible for free Medicare hospital insurance (Part A) can enroll in Medicare medical insurance (Part B) by paying a monthly premium.

If you are not eligible for free hospital insurance, you can buy medical insurance, without having to buy hospital insurance, if you are age 65 or older and you are:

- A U.S. citizen; or
- A lawfully admitted non-citizen who has lived in the U.S. for at least five years.

Part B covers certain medical items and services no matter how you get your Medicare health care. Costs for these services vary depending on the plan you choose.

Medicare Part B helps cover:

Ambulance Services: When you need to be transported to a hospital or skilled nursing facility, and transportation in any other vehicle would endanger your health.

Ambulatory Surgery Center: Facility fees are covered for approved services.

Blood: Pints of blood you get as an outpatient or as part of a Part B-covered service.

Bone Mass Measurement: To help see if you are at risk for broken bones. This service is covered once every 24 months (more often if medically necessary) for people with Medicare who meet certain medical conditions.

Cardiovascular Screenings: Every five years to test your cholesterol, lipid, and triglyceride levels to help prevent heart attack or stroke.

Chiropractic Services (limited): To correct a subluxation (when one or more of your bones of your spine moves out of position) using manipulation of the spine.

Clinical Laboratory Services: Including blood tests, urinalysis, some screening tests, and more.

Clinical Trials: To help doctors and researchers find better ways to prevent, diagnose, or treat diseases. Routine costs are covered if you take part in a qualifying clinical trial.

Colorectal Cancer Screenings: To help find precancerous growths, and help prevent or find cancer early, when treatment is most effective.

Diabetes Screenings: To check for diabetes.

Diabetic Self-Management: For people with diabetes. Your doctor or other health care provider must provide a written order.

Diabetic Supplies: Including glucose testing monitors, blood glucose test strips, lancet devices and lancets, glucose control solutions, and therapeutic shoes (in some cases). Syringes and insulin are only covered if used with an insulin pump or if you have Medicare prescription drug coverage.

Doctor Services: Doesn't cover routine physical exams except for the one-time "Welcome to Medicare" Physical Exam.

Durable Medical Equipment: Items such as oxygen, wheelchairs, walkers, and hospital beds needed for use in the home.

Emergency Room Services: When you believe your health is in serious danger, when every second counts. You may have a bad injury, sudden illness, or an illness that quickly gets worse.

Eyeglasses (limited): One pair of eyeglasses with standard frames after cataract surgery that implants an intraocular lens.

Flu Shots: To help prevent influenza or flu virus. This is covered once a flu season in fall or winter.

Foot Exams and Treatment: If you have diabetes-related nerve damage and/or meet certain conditions.

Glaucoma Tests: To help find the eye disease glaucoma. This is covered once every 12 months for people at high risk for glaucoma. Tests must be done by an eye doctor legally authorized to perform this service in your state.

Hearing and Balance Exam: If your doctor orders it to see if medical treatment is needed. Hearing aids and exams for fitting hearing aids aren't covered.

Hepatitis B Shots: To help protect people from getting Hepatitis B. This coverage is for people with Medicare at high or medium risk for Hepatitis B.

Home Health Services: Limited to reasonable and necessary part-time or intermittent skilled nursing care and home health aide services as well as physical therapy, occupational therapy, and speech-language pathology that are ordered by your doctor and provided by a Medicare-certified home health agency. Also, includes medical social services, other services, durable medical equipment, and medical supplies for use at home.

Kidney Dialysis Services and Supplies: Either in a facility or at home.

Mammograms (screening): To check women for breast cancer before they or their doctor may feel it. Preventative mammogram screenings are covered once every 12 months for all women with Medicare age 40 and older. Medicare covers one baseline mammogram for women between age 35 and 39.

Medical Nutrition Therapy Services: For people who have diabetes or renal disease (people who have kidney disease but aren't on dialysis or haven't had a kidney transplant, or for people who have kidney disease [but aren't on dialysis]) with a doctor's referral three years after a kidney transplant.

Mental Health Care (Outpatient): Certain limits and conditions apply.

Occupational Therapy: Services given to help you return to usual activities (such as bathing) after an illness.

Outpatient medical and Surgical Services and Supplies: For approved procedures.

Pap Test and Pelvic Exam (includes clinical breast exam): To check for cervical and vaginal cancers. Medicare covers these exams for women at low risk for cervical cancer every 24 months. These exams are covered once every 12 months for women at high risk for cervical and vaginal cancer, and those of child bearing age who have had an exam that indicated cancer or other abnormalities in the past three years.

Physical Exam (one-time "Welcome to Medicare" Physical Exam): A one-time review of your health, and education and counseling about preventative services, including certain screenings and shots.

Physical Therapy: Treatment of injuries and disease by mechanical means, such as heat, light, exercise, and massage.

Pneumococcal shot: To help prevent pneumococcal infections. Most people only need this preventative shot once in their lifetime.

Practitioner Services: Such as those provided by clinical social workers, physician assistants, and nurse practitioners.

Prescription Drugs: Limited, like certain injectable cancer drugs.

Prostate Cancer Screening: These tests help find prostate cancer.

Prosthetic/Orthotic items: Including arm, leg, back, and neck braces; artificial eyes; artificial limbs (and their replacement parts); breast prostheses (after mastectomy); prosthetic devices needed to replace an internal body part or function.

Second Surgical Opinions: Covered in some cases (and some third surgical opinions are covered) for surgery that isn't an emergency.

Smoking Cessation (counseling to stop smoking): Provided at any provider site if ordered by your doctor.

Speech-language Pathology Services: Treatment to regain and strengthen speech skills.

Surgical Dressings: For treatment of a surgical or surgically treated wound.

Telemedicine: Services in some rural areas, under certain conditions in a practitioner's office, a hospital, or a federally-qualified health center.

Tests: Including X-rays, MRIs, CT scans, EKGs, and some other diagnostic tests.

Transplant Services: Including heart, lung, kidney, pancreas, intestine, and liver transplants under certain conditions and in a Medicare-certified facility only. Bone marrow and cornea transplants (under certain conditions).

Travel (health care needed when traveling outside the USA): Limited.

Urgently Needed Care: To treat a sudden illness or injury that isn't a medical emergency.

For more information about Medicare Part B: call 1-800-MEDICARE.

Medicare Advantage plans (Part C)

If you have Medicare Parts A and B, you can join a Medicare Advantage (formerly Medicare + Choice) plan. With one of these plans, you do not need a Medigap policy, because Medicare Advantage plans generally cover many of the same benefits that a Medigap policy would cover, such as extra days in the hospital after you have used the number of days that Medicare covers.

Medicare Advantage plans include:

- Medicare managed care plans;
- Medicare preferred provider organization (PPO) plans;
- Medicare private fee-for-service plans; and
- Medicare specialty plans.

If you decide to join a Medicare Advantage plan, you use the health card that you get from your Medicare Advantage plan provider for your health care. Also, you might have to pay a monthly premium for your Medicare Advantage plan because of the extra benefits it offers.

People who become newly entitled to Medicare can enroll during their initial enrollment period or during the annual coordinated election period from November 15 – December 31 each year. There also will be special enrollment periods for some situations.

Medicare prescription drug plans (Part D)

Anyone who has Medicare hospital insurance (Part A), medical insurance (Part B) or a Medicare Advantage plan is eligible for prescription drug coverage (Part D). Joining a Medicare prescription drug plan is voluntary, and you pay an additional monthly premium for the coverage. You can wait to enroll in a Medicare Part D plan if you have other prescription drug coverage but, if you don't have prescription coverage that is, on average, at least as good as Medicare prescription drug coverage, you will pay a penalty if you wait to join later. You will have to pay this penalty for as long as you have Medicare prescription drug coverage.

77. What is Medigap?

Medigap is health insurance that supplements the benefits covered under Medicare. It also fills in some of the gaps left by Medicare, such as your deductible and coinsurance contributions. Sold by private insurance companies, Medigap insurance is offered in 10 different versions, Plans A through J, with each providing a different level of coverage.

Plan A covers the following basic benefits:

- Your co-insurance contribution for hospital visits that Medicare covers
- Full coverage for 365 additional hospital days for use after Medicare's coverage of 60 days is used up
- Your co-insurance contribution on doctors' bills that Medicare covers
- The first three pints of blood you may need in a year (Medicare pays for any additional blood)

Plans B through J cover the same basic benefits, plus some extra benefits that include different combinations of the following:

- The hospital deductible for visits that Medicare covers
- Daily coinsurance contribution for skilled nursing facility care
- The deductible for doctors' services that Medicare covers
- Eighty percent of emergency medical costs that are needed during the first two months of a trip outside the United States
- The difference between your doctor's fee and Medicare's allowance
- Custodial care, working together with Medicare's coverage
- Some prescription drug benefits
- Routine annual medical checkups and other preventive care

Some of the benefits NOT covered by Medigap include long-term nursing home care, and vision and dental care. Medigap will follow Medicare in excluding what is unnecessary or experimental.

If you are covered by your former employer's health insurance plan, you may not need Medigap. For the most part, that health insurance policy, combined with Medicare, is a complete coverage package.

78. What is Medicaid?

Everyone should learn about state laws concerning the way in which assets affect your ability to obtain Medicaid assistance.

Medicaid provides medical care to the poor, to children and to pregnant women living under the federal poverty level. It is funded jointly by the states and the federal government.

Medicaid was established in 1965, at the same time as Medicare, under Title XIX of the Social Security Act. It was designed to assist low-income families in providing health care for themselves and their children. It also covers certain individuals who fall below the federal poverty level. It covers hospital and doctor's visits, prenatal care, emergency room visits, drugs and other treatments.

Other people who are eligible for Medicaid include low-income children under age six, low-income pregnant women, Supplemental Security Income recipients, adopted or foster children, specially protected groups, children under age 19 whose family income is below federal poverty level, some Medicare beneficiaries and other groups, as determined by each state. Most families who receive welfare probably have a social worker assigned to them, and this person will usually advise a family on its Medicaid eligibility. Many doctors will also be able to inform their patients about Medicaid.

Medicaid can pay for a number of costs, including hospital bills, physician services, and long-term care. Medicaid is the single largest payer of nursing home bills in America and is the last resort for people who have no other way to finance their long-term care. Although the eligibility rules vary from state to state, federal minimum standards and guidelines must be observed.

In addition to you meeting your state's medical and functional criteria for nursing home care, your assets and monthly income must each fall below certain limits if you are to qualify for Medicaid. However, several assets (which may include your family home) and a certain amount of income may be exempt or not counted.

Although many people are ineligible for Medicaid when they first enter a nursing home, several states allow elders to enter and then spend down their income and assets on nursing home bills to become eligible. This can be a great advantage. On the downside, though, you may have to kiss your life savings good-bye.

That's where Medicaid planning comes in. In determining your eligibility for Medicaid, a state may count only the income and assets that are legally available to you for paying bills. You can make assets unavailable by giving them away or by holding them in certain trusts. However, in some cases, such transfers may create a period of ineligibility before you can collect Medicaid. So, to engage in proper Medicaid planning, you should consult an experienced elder law attorney.

Anyone feeling he or she may be eligible for Medicaid can contact the local department of human resources or the Internet for more information. Medicaid.gov is the official Web site and includes a wealth of information, as well as a toll-free number. As is the case when dealing with most federal programs, people are well-advised to seek out professional assistance and get as much information as possible about the program in order to receive the maximum benefit.

79. What is the Medicaid Waiver Program?

Home and community-based waivers (1915(c) are tools used by states to obtain federal Medicaid matching funds to provide long-term care to patients in settings other than institutions.

Waivers must be approved by Centers for Medicare/Medicaid Services (CMS) and are good for three years, after which they may be renewed every five years.

General Information:

Home and community-based care is increasingly being viewed as a preferable alternative to long-term institutional care.

Benefits the individual who may remain among friends and family;

Benefits the state because services may be provided for less than the cost of institutional care.

Goals:

To re-integrate individuals into their communities;

To ensure that quality services are delivered in the most effective and cost efficient manner through a coordinated system; and

To utilize program funds to leverage federal dollars and grants to support the long-term goals of the program.

Waiver Intent:

To provide Medicaid-eligible clients who meet nursing home level of care with long-term community-based services and supports necessary to live safely and independently in the community.

The program provides greater flexibility in serving beneficiaries since state plan Medicaid limits services to disabled adults.

80. What is Long Term Care Insurance?

In considering long-term care insurance policies various kinds of care are mentioned. Here are the most commonly used terms and their generally accepted meaning. Remember, the definitions given here can and often times are re-defined by carriers in their policy and given special meaning under a particular contract. It is important to read the fine print.

Skilled nursing care is needed for medical conditions that require care by specially trained nurses or therapists, who routinely are licensed by the state. This level of care is on the specific orders of a doctor who dictates the care to be provided and is usually required around the clock, 24 hours a day. It is the care given as part of a severe illness and can extend well after the severest level of an illness has passed. Skilled care can be provided in a person's home with help from practical, as opposed to registered, nurses.

Intermediate nursing care is associated with stable conditions that require daily supervision, but not around the clock care. It is less specialized than skilled nursing care, often involves more personal care and is supervised by registered nurses. Intermediate care is commonly needed for a matter of months and years.

Custodial care is intended to assist with daily living, which includes bathing, eating, dressing, and other routine activities. Special training or medical skills are not required. It is provided by unskilled nursing assistants in nursing homes, day care centers, and at home. It is often called personal care.

It is common for long-term care services to be provided in a person's home. It includes part-time skilled nursing care, practical nursing assistance, the services of a nurse's aide, physical or occupational therapy, homemaker assistants, and chore workers, who provide assistance with daily living activities.

The cost of long-term care is expensive, depending on the severity of a disability, the degree of care needed and where it is to be provided.

81. Who pays for long-term care?

The answer is simple: it comes from your cash and your assets, your family's assets and for those without assets it is paid by Medicaid programs administered by state government. More than half of nursing home bills are paid out-of-pocket by individuals and their families, and somewhat less than half are paid by state Medicaid programs. Insurance, and that includes Medicare, Medicare supplemental coverage and health insurance provided by employers, **does not pay for most long-term care expenses.**

Only in certain cases will Medicare cover the cost of some skilled nursing care in approved nursing homes or in your home, but there is no coverage for custodial or intermediate care or prolonged home health care.

82. Medicare does not offer long-term care as a benefit.

Medicare supplement policies are sold by private insurance companies and are offered to fill some of the gaps in Medicare coverage. Hospital deductibles and excess physicians' charges are routinely covered, but these policies do not cover long-term care expenses.

83. Who should buy long-term care insurance?

Long-term care insurance is not for everyone. For a limited population, long-term care policy makes sense as an affordable and worthwhile form of insurance. Buying long-term coverage should not cause financial hardship and force you to forego other financial needs. Whether long-term care insurance is appropriate requires a full financial analysis. Check with an Elder Law attorney or accountant.

Although the need for long-term care can arise gradually as a person ages and needs more and more assistance with activities of daily living, for most, a stroke or a heart attack will be the precipitating need. Those with acute illnesses may need nursing-home care for a matter of months, while others may need care for years.

84. Who offers long-term care policies?

Private insurance companies, both stock and mutual companies, sell long-term care policies through agents. Some sell coverage through the mail and others through senior citizen organizations, fraternal societies, continuing care retirement communities and other groups. Employers are beginning to offer long-term care policies to their employees, their employees' parents, and their retirees.

85. What are Veteran's benefits?

The Veterans Administration (VA) has various programs to help elderly and disabled veterans. In some cases, these VA benefits can supplement Medicaid benefits.

VA Medical Benefits. The medical benefits package is a health benefits plan available to enrolled veterans. Budgetary constraints make it necessary for the VA system to provide benefits based on a priority system. Upon enrollment, veterans are placed into priority groups, which then determine the types of services available to the veteran. Some of the benefits available include prescription drugs, home health services, and hospice care.

Under a rule adopted in 2002, the VA will grant a priority level to "severely disabled" veterans, even if the immediate health problem needing attention is unrelated to their military service.

VA Nursing Home Care. The VA has contracts with non-VA community nursing homes, such that veterans in the special entitlement category can receive care at VA expense. Eligibility for this benefit is extremely limited.

Aid and Attendance. A benefit provided by the VA that is often overlooked is called "Aid and Attendance." This benefit can be an excellent source of funds for long-term care for the elderly, either at home or in a facility.

It is available to certain wartime veterans or their dependents who are totally disabled because of a non-service connected condition, who are in financial need, and who need the aid and attendance of another person in order to avoid the hazards of the daily environment. Under this program, the amount received will vary, and it is an add-on to the basic pension program.

86. How can I find out what benefits I'm eligible for?

Go to: www.benefitscheckup.org

If you don't have a computer at home, visit the local library or a senior center that has computers, or ask a trusted friend or family member to help.

This web site can help people aged 55 and over and some younger people with Medicare find and get the benefits they are eligible for. Completing the questionnaire only takes a few minutes and it's free.

BenefitsCheckUp can find you programs that pay for:

- Prescription drugs
- Heating bills
- Housing/Rent
- Meal Programs
- Legal services
- Medical Costs
- In-home services.

It can also help you find:

- Tax relief
- Veteran's benefits
- Employment
- Volunteer Work
- Other helpful information and resources

You can also contact your local Area Agency on Aging.

87. Support Considerations

It is important to create a support team. Plan for times when you'll need help by making a list of people who are willing to help. Family members, friends and respite care workers can give you a break or help out when you can't be there.

On your list, include their phone numbers, the times they are available and the tasks they feel most comfortable doing.

88. What is the 211 Initiative?

2-1-1 is an easy to remember telephone number that, where available, connects people with important community services and volunteer opportunities. The implementation of 2-1-1 is being spearheaded by United Way and comprehensive and specialized information and referral agencies in states and local communities.

2-1-1 reaches approximately 196 million people (over 65% of the total U.S. population) in 41 states and the District of Columbia. Yet, millions of Americans still need to be connected. America needs 2-1-1 to be accessible nationwide. As the number of organizations providing specialized services is on the rise, people find it frustrating and confusing to access community services. 2-1-1 provides a one-stop service for vital information. While services that are offered through 2-1-1 vary from community to community, 2-1-1 provides callers with information about and referrals to human services for every day needs and in times of crisis. For example, 2-1-1 can offer access to the following types of services:

Basic Human Needs Resource: food banks, clothing, shelters, rent assistance, utility assistance.

Physical and Mental Health Resources: medical information lines, crisis intervention services, support groups, counseling, drug and alcohol intervention, rehabilitation, health insurance programs, Medicaid and Medicare, maternal health, children's health insurance programs.

Employment Support: unemployment benefits, financial assistance, job training, transportation assistance, education programs.

Support for Older Americans and Persons with Disabilities: home health care, adult day care, congregate meals, Meals on Wheels, respite care, transportation, and homemaker services.

Support for Children, Youth and Families: Quality childcare, Success by 6, after school programs, Head Start, family resource centers, summer camps and recreation programs, mentoring, tutoring, protective services.

Volunteer opportunities and donations.

89. Are there any community resources available to family caregivers?

Yes. It is important to make contact with community resources before you get started. They can offer a lot of help and support.

Resources are available to assist you in providing care and to give you respite from constant responsibilities of caregiving.

The local Area Agency on Aging (AAA) is one of the first resources you should contact when help is needed caring for an older person. Almost every state has one or more AAAs, which serve local communities, older residents, and their families. In a few states, the State Unit or Office on Aging serves as the AAA. Local AAAs are generally listed in the city or county government sections of the telephone directory under "Aging" or "Social Services."

> *Success is the sum of small efforts, repeated day in and day out.*
>
> – Robert Collier

Preparing the Home

Just how safe is your home? No matter how safe you feel, chances are, there are some precautions you can take to make your home safer and more secure. Every year thousand so of people are killed or injured in home accidents. However, many of these instances could have been prevented.

Adapting the home for a person who is partially or totally disabled can be a difficult process. The keys to making the home a safe home are awareness and precaution.

As the care-receiver changes so should the home environment.

90. What are some general safety tips I should consider?

- Emergency numbers and your address should be posted by each telephone.
- Ideally the home or living area should be on one level, and preferably the ground level. Stairs are a big danger for elderly people.
- Inside and outside door handles and locks are easy to operate.
- Doors have lever-action handles instead of round knobs.
- Install at least one stairway handrail that extends beyond the first and last steps.
- Remove any furniture that is not needed. Avoid clutter.
- All remaining furniture should be stable and without sharp corners to minimize the effects of a fall.
- Remove throw rugs, sharp objects and clutter.
- Place carpet or safety grip strips on stairs.
- Keep the layout of furniture and pathways the same.
- Make sure halls are 3' wide, 6'-8' high.
- Make sure chair seats are 20" high.
- Make sure all rooms have adequate lighting. In addition, use automatic night-lights in every room.
- Develop and practice a fire-escape plan. Keep clear fire escape routes.
- Place a smoke alarm in every bedroom and on every floor.
- Place a fire extinguisher in the kitchen and bedroom. Make sure it is in date.
- The water heater thermostat is set at 120 degrees F or lower.
- Medications are stored in a safe place.
- Keep several flashlights (and back-up batteries) on hand in case of a power failure. Do not use candles as they are a fire hazard.

91. What adaptations in the environment could make the home safer?

Consider the following:

- Lighting the home
  - window coverings
  - consistency of lighting within the home
  - increased lighting if necessary
- Memory aids
  - have a special place for reminders
  - a large calendar
  - a large clock
  - notes to remind about special events
  - use of timers
  - medication reminders

92. How can I make the bathroom safer?

The bathroom is the most likely area of a household where a person may fall. The following safety tips will help to avoid a fall or other possible accident:

- Install a nonskid mat or strips on the standing area in front of the bathtub or shower. Use rubber suction-grip mats, adhesive strips or anti-slip tub surface material to prevent slipping in tub. Keep them free of any soap scum build-up.
- Install grab bars on the walls by the bathtub and toilet to help with getting in or out of the tub/shower and on wall where extra support around toilet area. Permanently installed ones as well as removable clamp-on models are available. Never allow use of toilet paper holders, towel racks or wall mounted sinks for supporting one's weight.
- Consider purchasing a floor-to-ceiling vertical rod sometimes referred to as a safety pole that is easy to remove or relocate for use in strategic locations where extra support is needed.

- Firmly install towel bars and soap dish in the shower stall that are made of durable materials.
- Purchase a bathtub or shower seat made of sturdy molded plastic or padded vinyl for added comfort if preferred for those with poor standing balance or general weakness. They are available with or without backs, height adjustments, and heavy-duty models to accommodate greater weight capacities and slip-resistant rubber feet or foldaway portable models.
- Consider purchasing a transfer tub board that attaches to the tub to offer comfortable safe seating if less obtrusive device preferred, more portable, or may be a better fit in your existing bathtub.
- Purchase a transfer tub bench for those who have difficulty entering or exiting the tub. Transfer tub benches extend beyond the edge of the tub for those who have difficulty stepping over the tub wall safely. Check the weight capacity or additional six-leg support to accommodate user. Place bench so that two of the legs are on outside of tub and other two within tub. The user then sits safely on outside of the tub and slides to inside the tub while remaining seated on bench. Place these seats facing the faucet end of the tub
- Add hand held shower sprays for the user's convenience to help control water flow when seated on bath chairs and transfer benches. They easily attach to your existing shower arm, or can be attached with a diverter valve and used in conjunction with the existing showerhead for other family members.
- Purchase a raised toilet seat when the standard seat is too low to help those who have difficulty getting up and down from a regular toilet, bending or sitting. Look for those with safety features including brackets or locking clamps that stabilize the seat on the toilet rim.
- Bathroom flooring should be matte-finished, textured tile, or low pile commercial carpet. Do not use throw rugs or bath mats.
- Locate the light switch near the door.
- Make sure the bathroom has safe, supplemental heat source and ventilation system.
- Install outlets that are ground fault circuit interrupters (GFCI) to protect against electric shock.
- The bathroom door should open outward.

93. How can I make the bedroom safer?

To make the home safer and a more comfortable place to live, here are some things that can improve the safety of the bedroom area:

- Keep a lamp or flashlight within reach of your bed. Check the batteries periodically.
- Put a stable nightstand next to the bed. This provides a place for the older person's glasses and other necessary items within easy reach.
- Remove casters on beds, tables and chairs. Unintended movement of furniture used for support by the elderly person can result in a fall.
- Use a night-light to brighten the way to the bathroom at night.
- Make sure there is plenty of room to walk around the bed.
- Make sure there is a telephone in the room in case of an emergency
- For elderly who are smokers, arrange for a specific, safe place in the house where smoking is allowed. Discourage smoking in bed or while sitting on upholstered furniture.
- Draw up and practice an evacuation plan in case of fire or other emergency.
- Fix bed height so the older person can get on and off comfortably.
- See that storage spaces and needed items are within easy reach of the older person
- Place a sturdy chair with arms in bedroom where you can sit to dress.

94. What can I do to make the kitchen safer?

The kitchen is a busy area in the home and a likely place for an accident to occur. Simple ways to make your kitchen a safer place include:

- Use sturdy kitchen chairs with armrests and seats no higher or lower than 18 inches.
- Avoid chairs with wheels.
- Provide water-absorbent mats around the sink area, and use nonskid rugs, nonskid floor wax and nonskid-sole shoes.
- Make sure lighting is adequate to prevent tripping.
- Provide sturdy stepladders and caution against using kitchen chairs for standing on.

- Keep electrical cords, footstools and other low-lying objects out of kitchen walkways.
- Provide smoke detectors and carbon monoxide detectors.
- Keep a kitchen fire extinguisher or baking soda available to put out fires. Advise the use of nonflammable garments and avoidance of long-sleeved clothing that can get caught on appliances.
- Lighting of counter tops is enough for meal preparation.
- Oven controls are clearly marked and easily grasped.
- Flooring is not slippery and has a non-glare surface.
- When cooking, keep pan handles turned away from other burners and the edge of the range.
- Knives are kept in a knife rack or drawer. Never store knives loose in a drawer.
- Drawers and cupboards are kept closed.
- Grease or liquid spills are wiped up at once.

95. How can I keep the living room safer?

More than likely you will spend a lot of your time in the living room. Here are some safety tips to consider:

- Place electrical cords along walls, not under rugs, and away from traffic areas.
- Make sure chairs and couches are secure and sturdy.
- Clear passageways for traffic and make sure there is enough space to walk through the room.
- Make sure furniture that might be used for support when walking or rising is steady and does not tilt.
- Chairs and couches are not too low or too deep to get in and out of easily.
- Chairs and couches have full arms to aid in sitting or rising.
- The light switch is located near the entrance.

Equipment and Supplies

Having the right equipment and supplies can make caregiving tasks simpler, faster and more efficient. Assistive equipment is any kind of tool or device that can help simplify caregiving or make the environment safer for an ill, disabled, or elderly person. Equipment to consider:

- Bedside commode
- Hand-held shower
- Handrails
- Lift chair
- Ramp
- Raised commode seat
- Shower seat/bath bench
- Beds with special features that increase the person's ability to get in and out of bed
- Assistive telephones (for hearing-impaired and sight-impaired persons)
- Assistive stovetop burners (for sight-impaired persons)
- Walkers and canes
- Wheelchairs

There are many companies that provide adaptive equipment for communications, mobility, and recreation and offer adaptive clothing. There are many ways to obtain assistive equipment for the home. Talk with your physician or home health care provider about your particular needs and the best way to obtain assistive equipment. Contact agencies from the phonebook under Hospital Equipment and Supplies or under Medical Equipment and Supplies.

96. Are there any companies that lease medical equipment or do you have to purchase everything?

Yes, some companies offer a rental program. With proper doctor's orders (referrals) and documentation, some equipment is covered by Medicare and private insurance.

Medicare does not help pay for assistive devices, but does pay for durable medical equipment in some cases.

97. What is considered Durable Medical Equipment (DME)?

Durable medical equipment (DME) is equipment that is primarily and customarily used to serve a medical purpose, can withstand repeated use, and is appropriate for use in the home. Some examples of DME include hospital beds, walkers, wheel chairs and oxygen tents. Medical supplies of an expendable nature, such as bandages, rubber gloves and irrigating kits are not considered by Medicare to be DME.

Some local groups may allow you to borrow equipment for short-term use. Contact:

- Salvation Army
- Red Cross
- Home health care agencies
- National Easter Seal Society

- Faith-based groups and senior centers
- Your county Department on Aging
- Area Agencies on Aging

98. What general supplies will I need for caregiving?

Household Supplies:

- Linens: bed sheets, disposable underpads, pillows, blankets, towels, facecloths, pajamas
- Cleaning supplies: (along with usual detergents, bleach, deodorizers)
- Cooking & feeding utensils, ice cube trays, straws, feeding syringe
- Garbage bags, toilet paper, tissues, paper towels

Caregiving Supplies: *(may be available through a Home Care program)

- *Hospital bed with side rails, adjustable bedside table
- *Foam, air, sheepskin mattress
- *Commode (portable toilet)
- *Bedpan & urinal
- *Latex gloves, masks & plastic aprons
- *Disposable diapers/underpants & incontinence pads, panty liners
- *Wheelchair, walker or cane

Other General Supplies:

- Kidney basin
- Washing basin for bed baths
- 3 bins or baskets, one for linen & two for garbage
- Flashlight, nightlight
- Thermometer (oral and/or rectal)
- Watch or clock with a second hand
- Personal hygiene: toothbrush, combs, brush, nail clippers, shaving kit
- Hand cream or body lotion & talcum powder
- Vaseline, lotion
- Water jug
- Antiseptic or rubbing alcohol
- Antibacterial hand cleaner
- Bacteriostatic ointment
- Hydrogen peroxide
- Bandages, gauze pads, tape
- Cotton balls and swabs
- Container for disposing of syringes/needles
- Heating pad
- Ice bag
- Oral laxative
- First aid kit with manual
- Shower cap
- Ear thermometer

99. What medical equipment will I need to get?

The equipment you will need will depend on the care-receiver's medical condition. This equipment might include:

Bedroom:

- Hospital bed
- Alternating pressure mattress
- Egg-carton pad
- Portable commode chair
- Trapeze bar
- Transfer board
- Hydraulic lift
- Over the bed table
- Mechanical or electric chair lift
- Blanket support
- Urinal or bedpan

Bathroom:

- Elevated toilet seat
- Commode aid
- Toilet frame
- Grab bars for tub and shower
- Safety mat strips
- Hand-held shower hose
- Bath bench
- Bath transfer bench
- Bathtub safety rails

Mobility aids:

- Wheelchair
- Walker
- Electric scooter
- Crutches
- Cane
- Transfer board

Assistive devices:

Sight aids:

- Prism glasses
- Magnifying glasses
- Prescription glasses
- Braille books and signs
- Books on tape

Listening aids:

- Hearing aids
- Sound systems that amplify
- Telephone amplifiers
- Closed captioned TV

Eating aids:

- Spoons that swivel for those who have trouble with wrist movement
- Foam that can fit over utensils for easier gripping
- Plate guards for easier scooping, mugs with two handles, a cover, a spout and a suction base

Dressing aids:

- Button hooks to make buttoning easier, dressing sticks

Misc.

Equipment Cost-Comparison

For each item, compare the purchase price with the rental fee times months needed. Is the item covered by Medicare?

- bath stool
- bedpan
- bed safety accessories
- cane
- commode
- hospital bed
- mattress
- oxygen
- raised toilet seat
- special equipment
- trapeze
- walker
- wheelchair
- scooter
- other

Getting Through the Day

The duties of the caregiver usually change and increase over a period of time. One of the most difficult aspects of the caregiver role is that the job continues seven days a week, 24 hours a day. One way to help caregivers " get through the day" is to set up a care plan, develop a routine.

100. What is a Care Plan?

The Caregiver's Care Plan is very similar to the Nurse's Plan of Care and the Hospice Plan of Care. It is a daily record of the care and treatment of the care-receiver. It provides a record of events that assist everyone on the Care Team. It also allows another caregiver to take your place fairly easily.

101. Why should I use a written Care Plan?

With a written plan, you don't have to rely on your memory. A daily record will help both the caregiver and the care-receiver, and everyone on the Care Team. It will serve as a reference tool that can be reviewed as the care-receiver's needs or conditions change.

102. Setting up the Care Plan

For any Care Plan to work, the care-receiver should be included in every possible aspect of the planning process. This will not only assure that his or her dignity is respected, but also that the plan will be followed. This may be easier said than done! The care-receiver may not even be willing to admit that he/she needs help.

103. Where's the best place to start in developing a Care Plan?

By now the family should have determined who is going to be the primary caregiver. This person will have the main responsibility for the actual care.

Establishing a well thought-out Care Plan will help relieve stress for everyone involved. Many decisions will have to be made.

An evaluation of needs and activities can be done to assess and determine a baseline which will help determine the caregiver's duties.

Managing Feelings

Caregivers often experience a roller coaster of emotions — everything from guilt and resentment to hope and love. They often wonder if they will ever get their lives back. There are numerous emotional eruptions that come with caregiving of a loved one.

104. What can I do to manage my feelings?

Before you even start caregiving, set boundaries. Accept that there is a limit to what you can do as a caregiver. Recognize when you feel overwhelmed, and ask for help in caring for your loved one.

When caring for someone who is deteriorating, a caregiver often experiences many overwhelming feelings. It is natural to have emotional reactions to the challenges and responsibilities of your job. Caring for an aging person can bring out anger you may not even know you had. Suppressed anger can cause major problems in caring for family members. Often it is shown through impatience and irritability towards the care-receiver.

Even though there is no perfect formula for managing your feelings, it is imperative that you be aware of your feelings because they influence your behavior and judgment. Allow yourself to have the feeling. Remind yourself that such feelings are okay. Take a deep breath. What you do about the feeling is important.

105. What can I do to regain a good perspective?

Take a few deep breaths and exhale slowly. Focus on relaxing. Act instead of react. Take a moment to gain control of your feeling, and make a conscious decision of what you will do about it.

106. How important is communication style?

Communication style between the care-receiver and the caregiver is important. Effective expression of your feelings can release tensions and increase mutual understanding. Two ways to improve the situation:

1. Communicate. Express your feelings using "I" statements.
2. Avoid blaming statements which imply others are responsible for your feelings.

If you are unable to communicate your feelings, in order to relieve tension, then find another way to relieve tension. If you keep negative feelings bottled up, eventually it will lower your resistance to illness.

107. If I can't communicate my feelings, what are some other ways to relieve tension?

- Exercise. Go for a short, brisk walk, ride a bicycle, jump rope, aerobics.
- Punch a pillow.
- Clean the floor or bath tub.
- Cry or laugh. Even screaming releases tension. This doesn't mean should scream "at" someone. Find a private place to scream (alone in your car or in a basement closet) where you won't scare others.
- Keep a journal or write a letter and then tear it up.
- Confide in a close friend who is a good listener.
- Join a support group.

108. Why does it seem like family dynamics are getting worse instead of better?

Many times unresolved family issues come to the surface in a caregiver/care-receiver relationship. Family members either act as sources of support or sources of additional stress. Some family members find it easier to offer financial support rather than emotional support.

109. Why do I feel guilty?

Many caregivers do not know why they feel guilty. However, they can describe family conflicts, difficulties in making decisions, not knowing how else to help and host of other feelings and situations.

To begin to address this problem, substitute the word "disappointed" for "guilty". Almost everyone is familiar with disappointment. Disappointment can be shared, but guilt belongs only to you. It can quickly become a heavy burden.

110. What is elder abuse?

Elder abuse is doing something or failing to do something that results in harm to an elderly person or puts a helpless older person at risk of harm. This includes:

- **Passive and Active Neglect:** With passive and active neglect the caregiver fails to meet the physical, social, and/or emotional needs of the older person. The difference between active and passive neglect lies in the intent of the caregiver. With active neglect, the caregiver intentionally fails to meet his/her obligations towards the older person. With passive neglect, the failure is unintentional; often the result of caregiver overload or lack of information concerning appropriate caregiving strategies.
- **Physical Abuse:** Physical abuse consists of an intentional infliction of physical harm of an older person. The abuse can range from slapping an older adult to beatings to excessive forms of physical restraint (e.g. chaining).
- **Material/Financial Abuse:** Material and financial abuse consists of the misuse, misappropriation, and/or exploitation of an older adults material (e.g. possessions, property) and/or monetary assets.
- **Psychological Abuse:** Psychological or emotional abuse consists of the intentional infliction of mental harm and/or psychological distress upon the older adult. The abuse can range for insults and verbal assaults to threats of physical harm or isolation.
- **Sexual Abuse:** Sexual abuse consists of any sexual activity for which the older person does not consent or is incapable of giving consent. The sexual activity can range from exhibitionism to fondling to oral, anal, or vaginal intercourse.
- **Violations of Basic Rights:** Violations of basic rights is often concomitant with psychological abuse and consists of depriving the older person of the basic rights that are protected under state and federal law ranging from the right of privacy to freedom of religion.
- **Self Neglect:** The older person fails to meet their own physical, psychological, and/or social needs.

111. Why does elder abuse occur?

It can occur as a result of caregiver stress, impairment of the care-receiver, cycle of violence, or personal problems of abusers. Call information for your State Elder Abuse Hotline.

112. What can I do to prevent elder abuse?

It is imperative that you are aware of and deal with stress. You can do that by:

- Eating properly and getting enough sleep and exercise.
- Taking time to get away.
- Utilizing available family, friends or paid help.
- Scheduling visitors at different times to maximize the

time you can be relieved of caregiving responsibilities.
- Looking for positive experiences in caregiving.
- Maintaining a good sense of humor.
- Using community resources for information and support.
- Seeking assistance with difficult situations and behaviors — knowing what to expect helps.
- Joining a support group.
- Arranging for a comprehensive assessment to get specific recommendations.

113. What is the difference between loss, grief, and mourning?

Loss is unwanted change-something or someone has been taken from us. Grief is the internal response to loss and is most often characterized by anger, fear, sadness, and emptiness. Mourning is the external response to loss characterized by crying, yelling, forgetting, confusion or irritability.

The collective weight of losses that have accumulated over a lifetime, can burden the elderly in powerful and painful ways. When seniors lose their valued roles and behaviors, they grieve. They grieve spouses, parents, siblings and friends who have died. They grieve lost opportunities. They can grieve their lost hope for the future.

114. How do I manage feelings of grief and loss?

It is important to realize the grieving process is something that both you and the care-receiver will experience. Based on the studies of Elizabeth Kubler-Ross, caregiver grief has similar stages to those of other grief experiences. Be aware of the five stages of caregiver grief:

- Denial: not believing the diagnosis, pretending everything will be fine.
- Anger: which may be directed anywhere (at care-receiver, family members, God).
- Bargaining: searching for new therapies, new opinions.
- Depression; as the care-receiver declines the caregiver may experience physical illness, despair, and social isolation.
- Acceptance; living each day as well as possible, knowing that the death of a loved is imminent.

115. How can I help the care-receiver go through the stages of grief when facing death?

Here are some things you can do to make the process easier:

- Let your care-receiver know how proud you are of his/her accomplishments.
- Let him/her know how much you will miss him/her. People who feel they lived successfully may die more peacefully.
- If applicable, make use of comprehensive care and support offered by hospice.
- Offer some of his/her favorite things: smells, touches, music.
- Reminiscence about good times.
- Call other relatives and friends and give them a chance to visit.
- Request visits from clergy or spiritual counselors.

116. How can I heal myself following a loss?

Give yourself time to adjust. Be gentle with yourself and others while remembering that your behavior reflects your needs.

It is important to ask for help and support from family and friends while setting boundaries that honor your well being. Live in the present. Recognize your limitations of patience and endurance.

Stay physically, mentally, emotionally, and spiritually fit.

Taking Care of Yourself While Caregiving

It is as important for the well being of care-receivers that caregivers attend to their own needs, in addition to those of the care-receiver. It is important that you maintain your health and well being.

You owe it to yourself to find time for you. Without it, you may not have the mental strength to deal with all of the emotions you experience as a caregiver, including guilt and anger. Give yourself permission not to be perfect.

117. What are the signs of stress?

Signs of stress may include:

- Denial — about the illness or condition and its effect on the person who's been diagnosed.
- Anger — at the person who is ill or others: that no effective treatments or cures currently exist, and that people don't understand what's going on.
- Social withdrawal — from friends and activities that once brought pleasure.
- Anxiety — about facing another day and what the future holds.
- Depression — begins to break your spirit and affects your ability to cope. Exhaustion -- makes it nearly impossible to complete necessary daily tasks.
- Sleeplessness — caused by a never-ending list of concerns.
- Irritability — leads to moodiness and triggers negative responses and reactions.
- Lack of concentration — makes it difficult to perform familiar tasks.
- Health problems — begin to take their toll, both mentally and physically.

It is important to realize that the signs of stress differ, as each person has a somewhat unique way of responding and coping. Learn to identify your own signs of stress.

118. What are ways to reduce caregiver stress?

Even with conscious efforts taken to take care of physical and emotional needs, caregivers can still experience excessive stress.

- Set realistic expectations for yourself.
- Talk to someone who will listen. Share information and feelings with others.
- Get help-don't try to do everything by yourself.
- Educate yourself about caregiving
- Accept your feelings.
- Be positive.
- Look for humor.
- Take care of yourself.
- Take one day at a time-enjoy each day.
- Get help.

119. What are the greatest needs of caregivers?

Two of the greatest needs of caregivers are information and assistance.

120. What is respite care?

Respite care is temporary care given by another in place of the primary caregiver so the primary caregiver can take a break.

121. How important is respite care?

It is important in that it reduces the incidence of caregiver burnout.

122. How can a caregiver support group help me?

A support group is one way to share your feelings or troubles. In most support groups, you'll talk about your problems and listen to others talk; you'll not only get help, but you'll be able to help others, too. Most important, you'll find out that you're not alone.

www.MeAndMyCaregivers.com

For stress relief, visit our Caregiving Community and click on the Unwind Here icon.

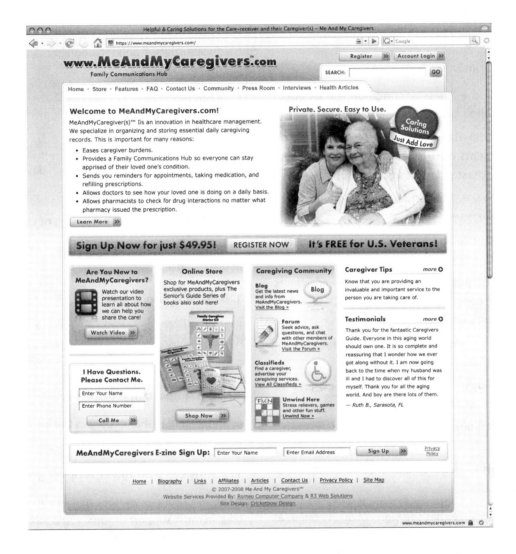

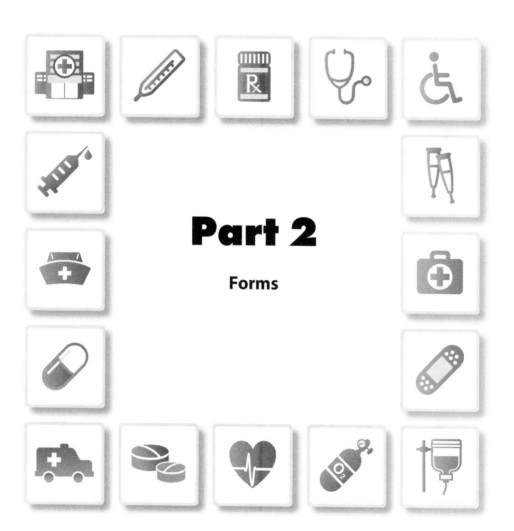

Part 2

Forms

How To Use The Forms

The purpose of the forms is to help both the care-receiver (the person who receives the care) and the caregiver record daily information that may be helpful to everyone on the caregiving team. Make copies of the forms and build your own caregiving organizer. Keep the daily records in a binder so they may be reviewed as needs and conditions change.

Your organizer will enhance communication between you, the doctors, and others on the care team.

Keep the binder in a prominent location near the care-receiver and/or caregiver, at all times. The caregiver will keep the records up-to-date. Take the binder to all medical appointments.

Checklists and Filling in the Forms

1. Getting Started Checklist .... Page 53

This is a general list that should be reviewed early on in the caregiving process.

2. Budget Worksheet .... Page 54

3. Valuable Records Checklist .... Page 55

Use this checklist to help the care-receiver keep track of valuable records. Be sure to store this list in a safe place since it contains valuable, personal, and private information.

4. General Care Evaluation .... Page 59

Complete the worksheet.

5. Personal Care Checklist .... Page 60

Complete the worksheet.

6. Release of Information and Consent Form .... Page 62

If you are a family caregiver, don't assume you automatically have rights to the care-receiver's information. To access another adult's information, have the care-receiver submit written authorization to his/her doctors and healthcare facilities.

In cases of lengthy or permanent incapacity, a legal guardian for the care-receiver may be appointed through court proceedings. When incapacity is anticipated, the care-receiver may grant power of attorney.

Use this form for release of information and consent in conjunction with doctors, agencies, family members, financial institutions, and other individuals for the purpose of helping the care-receiver to locate, receive, and monitor services and benefits to which he/she may be entitled.

7. In Case of Emergency .... Page 63

This form contains the care-receiver's emergency information. Keep it up-to-date. Make two copies. They should be the first two pages in your Organizer binder. In case of an emergency, tear out the first page and hand it to the paramedic or ER doctor. Take the complete binder with you to the hospital.

8. Emergency Wallet Card .... Page 64

This is a portable File of Life™-type card. Keep it up to date. Keep a legible copy in your wallet at all times.

9. Living Will Directive .... Page 65

Every state in the United States permits some form of Living Will Directive or Advance Health Care Directive, either by statute or judicial decision. Each state, however, has a different statute or case law that allows it. The Living Will form included in this publication should be recognized in most all states. Some states, however, have unique laws that require the use of a specific form. Additionally, state laws change from time-to-time, and sometimes new requirements are created. You should check the particular requirements of your state periodically to make sure the terms of your Living Will are enforceable. CONSULT WITH AN ATTORNEY TO REVIEW YOUR LIVING WILL.

10. Health Care Proxy and Durable Power of Attorney for Health Care.................................Page 67

Every state in the United States permits some form of Living Will or Advance Health Care Directive, either by statute or judicial decision. Each state, however, has a different statute or case law that allows it. The Health Care Proxy and Durable Power of Attorney for Health Care form included in this publication should be recognized in most all states. Some states, however, have unique laws that require the use of a specific form. Additionally, state laws change from time-to-time, and sometimes new requirements are created. You should check the particular requirements of your state periodically to make sure the terms of your Living Will are enforceable. CONSULT WITH AN ATTORNEY TO REVIEW YOUR HEALTH CARE PROXY AND DURABLE POWER OF ATTORNEY FOR HEALTH CARE

11. Prehospital Do Not Resuscitate (DNR) Form...Page 69

In the hospital, DNR orders are part of your medical records and all medical professionals should be aware of them. For out-of-hospital occurrences, say in the home, a proscribed placard may need to be displayed, to ensure your wishes are adhered to. Check your state regulations. In an emergency situation, EMS staff members do not have time to look for, or to evaluate different types of documentation. There is a possibility they may not acknowledge your directive, unless it is in plain sight.

12. Personal Information..Page 70

This form is straightforward. Interview the care-receiver and fill in the blanks. This is a good way to get to know the care-receiver.

13. Care Team Contact Information..Page 71

Fill in the blanks. Under specialists, start with the specialists the care-receiver sees most frequently.

14. My Health Now...Page 72

This form is designed to get a snapshot view of the care-receiver's current health. List the ailment/condition, the prescribed care plan or treatment, the name of the prescribing doctor, and any other information, such as things to keep an eye out for. If and when a new condition arises, simply add it to the bottom of the list. If a condition or ailment goes away, cross it off the list.

15. My Past Health History...Page 73

This form is designed record information about your past health.

16. My Daily Living Routine and Activities...Page 74

Fill in the blanks. You can use this information as a baseline of the care-receiver's condition. If there is a significant change in activities and preferences this may be valuable information for the doctor.

17. Leisure and Recreational Activities...Page 76

Interview the care-receiver and fill in the blanks.

18. Calendar...Page 77

Start by filling in the days, month and year. Write down the expiration dates of all medications. Add social and medical appointments. Review the calendar before your shift. If the care-receiver is having a special day, be sure to make a note of it on the calendar. Keep previous month's calendars in the back of the binder.

19. Questions for the Doctor . . . . Page 78

If you or the care-receiver has a question for the doctor, write it down here. Be sure to include the date. After you speak with the doctor, be sure to write down his/her response and action plan.

20. Lab Tests, X-Rays & Hospital Visits . . . . Page 79

This form is for keeping track of the care-receiver's lab tests, x-rays, or diagnostic tests. Also, include any hospitalizations, emergency room, or urgent care visits. Be sure to record follow-up visits on the monthly calendar. When this form is full store old copies in the back of the binder.

21. Reminders/Shopping List . . . . Page 80

This is a good place to keep a list of "things to do". When the task has been completed, scratch it off the list. If friends ask if there is anything they can do to help, refer to your list!

22. My Medications . . . . Page 81

This is an important form! Each month the medication information should be updated. Cross off any medications that the care-receiver discontinues. Be sure to add any new medications to the list. Record the refill date on the calendar. Keep the previous month's records in the back of the binder.

23. Daily Logs . . . . Page 82

You are going to need lots of copies of these forms, one for each day. Fill in the date. On an hourly basis, record if the care-receiver takes any medications, eats or drinks anything. List any activities, including bathroom visits, and naps or sleep. Initial each line. At the bottom of the page, there is a place to record any care-receiver or caregiver questions. This information could be important to the next caregiver, family member or doctor.

24. Respite Caregiver Checklist . . . . Page 84

This form will help the respite caregiver get a snapshot view of the care-receiver's condition. Be sure to go over each item with the respite caregiver.

25. End-of-Life Issues Checklist . . . . Page 86

Talk with the care-receiver to find out his/her end-of-life issues preferences.

Getting Started Checklist

Caregiving

- Learn as much as you can about caregiving. Attend caregiver training.
- Develop knowledge of community resources.
- Develop caregiving care plan, including alternate plans for care of the patient in the event of your illness.
- Make the home safe for the patient (accident-proofing).
- Determine what you are emotionally/physically able to do. Arrange for additional assistance through family, volunteers, respite care (home health care, adult day care or short-term respite care in a facility).
- Identify/attend local support group meetings.
- Schedule regular medical care for yourself, reporting any changes in your health to your physician.

Medical

- Get a complete diagnostic work-up on the care-receiver. Discuss with the physician regarding what is happening and what to expect.
- Schedule routine visits for both care-receiver and caregiver. Determine care-receiver's current level of functioning.
- Know care-receiver medical history, medications and dosages.

Legal

- Determine if the care-receiver needs assistance to manage his or her legal/financial affairs.
- Consult an Elder Law Attorney knowledgeable in issues such as Medicaid, Medicare, Guardianship, Estate Planning, Trusts and Advanced Directives. Contact attorney for advice regarding:
  - Durable Power of Attorney
  - Durable Power of Attorney for Health Care
  - Living Will
  - Will
  - Trusts
  - Guardianship
- If documents have been prepared previously, know location and check that they are up to date with current state laws.

Financial

- Someone should assume the responsibility for: Checking and Savings Account
- Other Assets (Money Market, Stocks, Bonds, CDs)
- Real Estate and other property (location of deeds)
- Safety Deposit Box-- Co-signer for box access (location of box and keys)
- Security Box or home safe (location and key combination.)
- Review and determine the location of all insurance policies (Medical, Disability, House, Car, Long Term Care, Life Insurance, VA.)
- Check for Waiver of Premium Clause on insurance policies.
- Investigate care-receiver's eligibility for financial assistance programs.
- Determine the amount and source of all monthly income.
- If the care-receiver is receiving Social Security, do you want to be designated as the Representative Payee?

Other

- Driving (You must judge when the patient can no longer safely operate a motor vehicle.)
- ID Bracelet for Alzheimer's disease patient, particularly if wandering becomes a problem.
- Develop safety plan if getting lost or wandering is an issue of the care-receiver.
- Develop an emergency back-up plan. Appoint someone who will know where your important papers are located.

Budget Worksheet

Fixed Expenses	Planned	Actual
Rent or Mortgage Payments		
Child Care		
Debt Repayment		
Allowance for Self		
Allowance for Others		
Car Payment		
Other		
Other		
Savings for Retirement		
Total Fixed Expenses:		

Flexible Expenses	Planned	Actual
Food at Home		
Personal Care		
Telephone		
Clothing		
Medicine		
Gasoline/Bus		
Laundry/Dry Cleaning		
Household Supplies/Home Care		
Food Away from Home		
Other		
Other		
Utilities		
Total Flexible Expenses:		
Total Fixed Expenses:		
Total Expenses:		

VALUABLE RECORDS CHECKLIST

Use this checklist to help you keep track of your valuable records. Be sure to store this list in a safe place since it contains some of your most valuable personal information.

Personal Records of: _____

Maiden or Other Names: _____

Date of Birth: _____

FAMILY	Name	Address	Phone	E-mail
Spouse/Partner:				
Children:				
Siblings:				

IDENTIFICATION RECORDS	Number/Notes	Location
Social Security Card:		
Driver's License:		
Birth Certificate:		
Marriage License(s):		
Divorce Record(s):		
Spouse's Death Certificate:		
Adoption Certificate:		
Naturalization Papers:		

MILITARY RECORDS	Number/Notes	Location
Military ID:		
Discharge Certificate:		

HEALTH CARE RECORDS	Description	Location
Personal Medical Info:		
List of Current Medications:		

IMPORTANT ADVISORS	Name	Phone	E-mail
Attorney:			
Executor/Personal Rep:			
Doctor(s):			
Religious Advisor:			
Accountant/Tax Advisor:			
Bank/Trust Officer:			
Health Insurance Agent:			
Auto Insurance Agent:			
Home Insurance Agent:			
Other:			

PHARMACY	Address	Phone	E-mail

VALUABLE RECORDS CHECKLIST

FINANCIAL RECORDS	Description	Location
Financial Assets Inventory		

FINANCIAL INFORMATION	Account Number	Institution
Checking Accounts:		
Savings Accounts:		
CDs/Savings Bonds:		

INVESTMENTS	Institution	ID Number	Beneficiary	Value
Stocks and Bonds:				
Shares of Mutual Funds:				
IRAs:				
Keogh Plans:				
401k Plans:				

SOURCES OF REVENUE	Description
Employer:	
Business or Self-employed:	
Retirement Plan:	
Pension Plan:	
Annuity Contracts:	
Military Retirement Benefits:	
Government Programs:	
Tax Refunds:	
Insurance Claims/Settlements:	
Other:	

REAL ESTATE OWNED	Description
Primary Residence:	
Secondary Residence:	
Vacation Property/Timeshare:	
Real Property:	
Vacant Land:	

PERSONAL PROPERTY OWNED	Description
Automobiles:	
Other Vehicles:	
Antiques:	
Collections:	
Jewelry:	

VALUABLE RECORDS CHECKLIST

INVENTORY OF MONEY OWED	Description
Mortgages:	
Home Equity Loans:	
Automobile Loans/Leases:	
Other Secured Loans:	
Business Loans:	
Unsecured Loans:	
Credit Card Debt:	

CREDIT CARDS	Account Number	In Name Of	Contact Phone Number

DEED LOCATIONS	Description	Location
Deed to House:		
Deeds to Other Properties:		
Automobile Titles:		
Loan Agreements:		
Tax Records:		

INSURANCE RECORDS	Policy Number	Name, Address, Phone	Beneficiary	Location
LIFE INSURANCE				
Group:				
Whole Life:				
Term Life:				
Universal Life:				
Other:				
HEALTH INSURANCE				
Major Medical Benefits:				
Health Insurance Supplement:				
Medigap Policy:				
Disability Insurance:				
Long Term Care:				
VEHICLE INSURANCE				
Automobiles:				
RVs:				
Campers:				
Boats:				
Airplanes:				
Other Vehicles:				
OTHER INSURANCE				
Homeowner's/Renter's:				
Liability:				
Personal:				
Business:				
Professional:				

VALUABLE RECORDS CHECKLIST

END-OF-LIFE PLANNING	Document Location
Last Will and Testament:	
Final Instructions/Personal Letter:	
Advance Medical Directives:	
Living Will:	
Durable Power of Attorney for Health Care:	
CPR Directives:	
Burial Policy/Ownership Certificate for Cemetery Plot:	

OTHER IMPORTANT DOCUMENTS	Document Location
Computer Passwords:	
Security Codes:	
Citizenship Papers:	
Bill(s) of Sale:	
Baptism Records:	
Diplomas:	
Household Inventory:	
Passport Papers:	
Power of Attorney:	
Education Records:	
Employment Records:	
Family History:	
Genealogy:	
Income Tax Records:	
Safe Deposit Box Inventory:	
Whom to Notify in Emergency:	

OTHER RECORDS	Document Location

www.MeAndMyCaregivers.com

General Care Evaluation

Housekeeping

_____ Needs help with all housekeeping chores.

_____ Does not participate in any housekeeping chores.

_____ Performs certain housekeeping chores satisfactorily.

_____ Maintains house in good order but requires help occasionally.

Food Preparation

_____ Needs help in preparing meals at all times.

_____ Prepares adequate meals with some help.

_____ Heats and serves meals prepared by others.

_____ Can prepare meals with no help.

Transportation

_____ Needs a companion to travel with.

_____ Arranges transportation (taxi, car) on his/her own.

_____ Cannot travel by bus.

_____ Drives own car.

Finances

_____ Cannot manage own money.

_____ Manages day to day expenses but needs help with major purchases and monthly bank reconciliation.

_____ Manages financial matters independently.

Telephone/Correspondence

_____ Can answer the phone but cannot dial out.

_____ Needs help in making calls or writing correspondence.

_____ Can use the phone and write letters without any help.

_____ Can use the computer.

Personal Care Checklist

Medications

_____ Cannot take medications without help.

_____ Needs to be reminded when to take medications.

_____ Does not need any help (when, how) in taking medication.

Physical Movement

_____ Needs help in moving around the house.

_____ Needs some kind of aid (wheelchair, cane, companion) when moving in or out the house.

_____ Does not need any assistance in walking or moving about.

Feeding

_____ Requires help in feeding self.

_____ Requires some help in feeding self with certain kinds of food.

_____ Can feed self without assistance.

Grooming

_____ Needs total grooming at all times.

_____ Needs help in grooming (remains well groomed after).

_____ Grooms self adequately but requires some help in using aids (shaver, hair dryer).

_____ Does not require any help.

Toileting

_____ Has no bowel control.

_____ Has no bladder control.

_____ Has bowel or bladder accidents once or twice a week.

_____ Needs to be reminded to use the toilet.

_____ Has no bowel or bladder difficulty.

Dressing

_____ Needs help in dressing or undressing.

_____ Dresses or undresses self with minimum assistance.

_____ Dresses or undresses self independently.

Personal Care Checklist, cont.

Bathing

_____ Cannot wash self or does not wash self.

_____ Can only wash face and hands.

_____ Needs help in getting in or out of bath tub.

_____ Needs help in getting in or out of shower.

_____ Can bathe, wash and clean self without help.

*** It is important to note the date when the care-receiver requires constant help in a task or activity which was not checked previously, as the Care Team may find the information useful in maintaining care.

Keep in mind that your evaluation of the care-receiver will change over time.

Release of Information and Consent Form

I, _____, hereby authorize

_____ to release and/or obtain information about me and/or from doctors, agencies, family members, financial institutions and other individuals as necessary for the purpose of helping me to locate, receive and monitor services and benefits to which I may be entitled. I further understand that I have the right to refuse to release information about me to specific individuals, agencies, and doctors.

I am aware that all information provided will be held private and confidential and that I may have access to the information about me.

This authorization will be in effect until _____.

_____ _____
Signature of Care-receiver/Patient   Signature of Witness

_____ _____
Social Security Number   Date of Signatures

Faxed copy of this form is an acceptable means of identification.

In Case of Emergency

Primary Care Doctor

Name: _____

Address: _____

Telephone Number(s): _____

Insurance: _____

Main Contact

Name: _____

Relationship: _____

Address: _____

City/State/Zip: _____

Home Phone: _____

Work Phone: _____

Cell Phone: _____

Secondary Contact

Name: _____

Relationship: _____

Address: _____

City/State/Zip: _____

Home Phone: _____

Work Phone: _____

Cell Phone: _____

Ambulance: _____

Hospital: _____

Medication Allergies: _____

Special Treatments: _____

Physical Aids (glasses, dentures, etc.): _____

Prosthesis: _____

Memory Loss/Dementia: _____

Family Members: _____

Neighbor/Friend: _____

Minister/Priest/Rabbi: _____

Organ Donor: ❏ Yes _____

❏ No

Living Will: ❏ Yes ❏ No

Location: _____

_____

_____

Do-Not-Resuscitate Order: ❏ Yes ❏ No

Location: _____

_____

Durable Power of Attorney for Health Care: ❏ Yes ❏ No

Location: _____

_____

Contact: _____

Emergency Wallet Card

(Keep up to date.)

Name:

Address:

Date of Birth:

EMERGENCY CONTACTS

Name:	Name:
Address:	Address:
Relation:	Relation:
Home Phone:	Home Phone:
Work Phone:	Work Phone:
Mobile:	Mobile:

FOLD

MEDICAL DATA

Last Updated:	Blood Type:

Primary Doctor/Phone:

Preferred Hospital:

Special Conditions/Remarks:

MEDICATION	DOSAGE	FREQUENCY
1.		
2.		
3.		
4.		
5.		
6.		
7.		
8.		
9.		
10.		

FOLD

Recent Surgery:	Date:
Recent Surgery:	Date:

Allergies:

Living Will   ❏ No   ❏ Yes   Location:

Durable Power of Attorney   ❏ No   ❏ Yes   Location:

DNR Form   ❏ No   ❏ Yes   Location:

Living Will Directive

I, _____, being of sound mind and at least 19 years old, and residing in the State of _____ hereby make the following wishes and directions known. It is my intention that this Living Will Directive be honored and followed by my family and attending physician(s) as the final expression of my legal right to refuse medical or surgical treatment and accept the consequences of such refusal. It is my intention that this advance directive constitute clear and convincing evidence of my wishes concerning medical treatment if I am unable to make or communicate my own health care decisions at that time. This Living Will Directive is intended to be valid in any jurisdiction in which it is presented and shall not be affected or revoked by my disability. I direct my attending physician and other health care providers, pursuant to the law applicable in the state whose law controls my medical treatment at that time, to withhold or withdraw treatment from me under the circumstances I have indicated below by my initials and/pr signature.

These directions may only be used if I am not able to speak for myself. If I am female and known to be pregnant, I do not want life-sustaining treatment and/or artificially provided food and hydration withheld or withdrawn (Notwithstanding any other provision in this Living Will) as long as it remains possible that the embryo/fetus will develop to the point of live birth. If my healthcare provider does not want to follow the directions in this document, he/she is directed to see that I get to a doctor or provider that will follow my directions. I consent to be given treatment that is necessary for my comfort or to alleviate my pain if it does not contradict any of my specific instructions below.

My specific instructions are as follows (initial those statements you wish to be included in the document and cross through those statements which do not apply):

a. If my death from a terminal condition is imminent and even if life-sustaining procedures are used there is no reasonable expectation of my recovery—

_____ I direct that my life not be extended by life-sustaining procedures, including the administration of nutrition and hydration artificially.

_____ I direct that my life not be extended by life-sustaining procedures, except that, if I am unable to take food by mouth, I wish to receive nutrition and hydration artificially.

_____ I direct that, even in a terminal condition, I be given all available medical treatment in accordance with accepted health care standards.

b. If I am in a persistent vegetative state, that is if I am not conscious and am not aware of my environment nor able to interact with others, and there is no reasonable expectation of my recovery within a medically appropriate period—

_____ I direct that my life not be extended by life-sustaining procedures, including the administration of nutrition and hydration artificially.

_____ I direct that my life not be extended by life-sustaining procedures, except that if I am unable to take in food by mouth, I wish to receive nutrition and hydration artificially.

_____ I direct that I be given all available medical treatment in accordance with accepted health care standards.

c. I have the following additional instructions (write "none" on each line, if no additional instructions are given:

_____

_____

_____

_____

Living Will Directive

The above **Living Will Directive** constitutes my desires and instructions in the event I become ill and am unable to speak for myself, and I have placed my initials where indicated above, and my signature below, in the presence of witnesses, in order to express those intentions and desires by clear and convincing evidence. I have signed this document after careful consideration and I state that it is in accordance with my strong convictions and beliefs. I want the wishes and directions here expressed carried out to the full extent permitted by law. Insofar as any of my instructions are not legally enforceable, I hope that those who are lawfully responsible for my medical care will regard themselves as morally bound by these provisions.

Your signature: _____

The declarant who signed above in my presence has personally been known to me and I believe him/her to be of sound mind and free of duress when he/she executed the foregoing instrument. I did not sign the declarant's signature above for or at the direction of the declarant, and I am not the health care proxy named above. I am at least 21 years of age and am not related to the declarant by blood, adoption, marriage, nor am I entitled to, or have any present or inchoate claim against, any portion of the estate of the declarant according to the laws of intestate succession of the in which this is being executed or under any testamentary will of the declarant or codicil thereto as of the date of declarant's signature. Neither am I directly responsible (financial or otherwise) for declarant's medical care. I am not the declarant's attending physician, an employee of the attending physician, or an employee of the health or care facility in which the declarant is a patient. I am not prohibited by any existing law from being a witness.

Name of first witness: _____

Signature: _____ Date signed: _____

Name of second witness: _____

Signature: _____ Date signed: _____

Acknowledgment

On the _____ day of _____, 20____, before me personally came _____, known to me to be the person who executed for forgoing Living Will Directive, and who acknowledged that he/she executed the same, and placed his/her initials to the same in the presence of the witnesses indicated thereupon.

NOTARY SEAL

_____
Notary Public Signature

State of _____

My Commission Expires: _____

Health Care Proxy and Durable Power of Attorney for Health Care

I, _____, being of sound mind at least 19 years old, and residing in the State of _____ hereby make the following Health Care Proxy and Durable Power of Attorney for Health Care. By executing this document, I intend to appoint the person(s) named herein as my agent to make medical decisions for me if I become too sick to speak for myself.

PLACE YOUR INITIALS BY ONLY ONE ANSWER:

I want the person listed below to be my health care proxy. I have talked with him/her about my wishes. I understand and direct that if there is a conflict between my health care proxy's decision and any Living Will which I have executed in writing, my Living Will shall take precedence.

First choice for proxy: _____

Relationship to me: _____

Address: _____

City, State, Zip: _____

Home Telephone: _____ Cell phone: _____

If the person named above is not able, not willing, or not available to be my health care proxy, this is my next choice. I have talked with him/her about my wishes that he/she act as my health care proxy if the person named above is unwilling or unable to do so. I understand and direct that if there is a conflict between my health care proxy's decision and any Living Will which I have executed in writing, my Living Will shall take precedence.

Second choice for proxy: _____

Relationship to me: _____

Address: _____

City, State, Zip: _____

Home Telephone: _____ Cell phone: _____

Instructions to Proxy: Place your initials by either "Yes" or "No"

I want my proxy to make all decisions about my medical care, including whether to give me artificially provided food and hydration if I am terminally ill or injured or permanently unconscious, notwithstanding what is set forth in any Living Will that I have executed.

_____ Yes _____ No

I want my proxy to make all decisions about my medical care, except that he/she must strictly follow my directions in any Living Will that I have executed about whether to withhold or terminate medical treatment, and/or whether to give me artificially provided food and hydration, if I am terminally ill or injured or permanently unconscious.

_____ Yes _____ No

Health Care Proxy and Durable Power of Attorney for Health Care

My above-named Health Care Proxy shall be my agent for all matters relating to health care. This Health Care Proxy and Durable Power of Attorney for Health Care is to remain in effect after my death for my agent to make decisions regarding autopsy, organ donation, or disposition of any remains. If I am unconscious, comatose, senile or otherwise unable to communicate, my agent may do what he/she deems necessary consistent with the terms of this Health Care Proxy and Durable Power of Attorney for Health Care, including but not limited to:

Strike out any Power you do not wish to give to your Health Care Proxy.

1. Employing and discharging medical, social service, and other support personnel responsible for my care; contracting on my behalf for any health care related service or facility for my care, without my agent incurring personal financial liability for such contracts;
2. Granting any waiver or release from liability required by any hospital, physician or other health care provider;
3. Having access to medical records and information to the same extent I am entitled to, and releasing my medical information to third parties, including, but not limited to hospitals, medical clinics and insurance companies;
4. Summoning emergency medical personnel and seek emergency treatment for me, or choosing not to do so, as my agent may deem appropriate given any instructions regarding such care that are expressed in any Living Will that I have executed and any medical status at the time of the decision.;
5. Pursuing any legal action in my name, at the expense of my estate, to force compliance of my wishes as determined by my agent, or to seek actual or punitive damages for the failure to comply;

All of my agent's actions under this Health Care Proxy and Durable Power of Attorney for Health Care during any period when I am unable to make or communicate health care decisions or when there is uncertainty whether I am dead or alive shall have the same effect on my heirs, devisees and personal representatives as if I were alive, competent, and acting for myself.

Your signature: _____ Date: _____

I, _____, am willing to serve as Health Care Proxy for the person who executed the foregoing Health Care Proxy and Durable Power of Attorney for Health Care and will follow the instructions above to the best of my ability.

Signature: _____ Date: _____

I, _____, am willing to serve as Health Care Proxy if the first choice cannot serve and will follow the instructions above to the best of my ability.

Signature: _____ Date: _____

Emergency Medical Services
Prehospital Do Not Resuscitate (Dnr) Form

An Advance Request to Limit the Scope of Emergency Medical Care

I, _____ request limited emergency care as herein described.
(Print patient's name)

I understand DNR means that if my heart stops beating or if I stop breathing, no medical procedure to restart breathing or heart functioning will be instituted.

I understand this decision will not prevent me from obtaining other emergency medical care by pre-hospital emergency medical care personnel and/or medical care directed by a physician prior to my death.

I understand I may revoke this directive at any time by destroying this form.

I give permission for this information to be given to the prehospital emergency care personnel, doctors, nurses or other health personnel as necessary to implement this directive.

I hereby agree to the "Do Not Resuscitate" (DNR) order.

_____   _____
(Patient/Surrogate signature)   (Date)

_____
(Print Surrogate's name)   (Relationship to the patient)   (Surrogate's phone number)

I affirm that this patient/surrogate is making an informed decision and that this directive is the expressed wish of the patient/surrogate. A copy of this form is in the patient's permanent medical record.

In the event of cardiac or respiratory arrest, no chest compressions, assisted ventilations, intubation, defibrillation, or cardiotonic medications are to be initiated.

_____   _____
(Physician signature)   (Date)

_____
(Print Name)   (Medical License Number)   (Phone number)

(THIS FORM WILL NOT BE ACCEPTED IF IT HAS BEEN AMENDED OR ALTERED IN ANY WAY)

Personal Information

My name is _____.

I like to be called _____.

I am _____ years old.

My spouse's name is _____.

My companion or roommate's name is _____.

I have _____ children:

Name	Where They Live/Phone Number

I have _____ siblings:

Name	Where They Live/Phone Number

I have _____ grandchildren and _____ great-grandchildren.

I have _____ cat(s) and _____ dog(s). Their names are: _____
_____.

My favorite hobbies are (or have been): _____
_____
_____.

Care Team Contact Information

Care-receiver Name: _____

Date of Birth: _____/_____/_____

Health Insurance: _____ Phone Number: _____

Policy Number: _____

	Name/Specialty	Phone Number
Primary Care Doctor		
Specialist		
Specialist		
Specialist		
Specialist		
Specialist		
Specialist		
Specialist		
Specialist		
Specialist		
Specialist		
Pharmacy		
Pharmacy		
Hospital		
Hospital		
Caregiver Agency		

My Health Now

Date:			
Ailment/Condition	**Care Plan**	**Doctor**	**Other Info**

My Past Health History

Major Illnesses (date, illness type, treatment — list most recent first)

1.
2.
3.
4.
5.

Hospitalizations (date, reason, treatment — list most recent first)

1.
2.
3.
4.
5.

Surgeries/Procedures (date, type, outcome — list most recent first)

1.
2.
3.
4.
5.

Chronic Diseases (type, when diagnosed, treatment)

1.
2.
3.
4.
5.

Relevant Family Health History (include spouse or companion):

Name/Relation	Condition	Age Attained/Death

My Daily Living Routine and Activities

Personal Care

Grooming and Dressing: _____
_____
_____

Bathing: _____
_____
_____

Toileting: _____
_____
_____

Sleep Preferences

Wake-Up: _____
_____

Naps: _____
_____

Bed-time: _____
_____

Notes: _____
_____

Eating Habits

Special Diet or Restrictions: _____
_____
_____

Likes and Dislikes: _____
_____

Chewing and Swallowing Problems: _____
_____

Texture Preferences: _____
_____

My Daily Living Routine and Activities, cont.

Eating Habits, cont.

Food Allergies: _____
_____
_____

Favorite Snacks: _____
_____
_____

Special Habits: _____
_____
_____

Preferences of Eating Times: _____
_____

Exercise/Mobility

Problems in and/or outside the home: _____
_____
_____

Walking: _____
_____

Stairs: _____
_____

Barriers: _____
_____

Wheelchair, Walker, Cane: _____
_____

Additional: _____
_____

Other Preferences: _____
_____
_____

Leisure and Recreational Activities

Pets: _____

_____

_____

Music: _____

_____

Radio: _____

_____

Favorite TV Shows: _____

_____

Books: _____

_____

Playing Cards: _____

_____

Short Walks: _____

_____

Naps: _____

_____

Conversation About: _____

_____

Newspapers: _____

_____

Room Temperature Preferences: _____

Lighting Preference: _____

Goals (health, recreation, social, etc.): _____

_____

_____

_____

_____

_____

_____

_____

My Calendar

Month: _____ Year: _____

Sunday	Monday	Tuesday	Wednesday	Thursday	Friday	Saturday

Questions for the Doctor

Doctor's Name: _____

Date: _____

Question: _____
_____

Response: _____
_____
_____

Action Plan: _____
_____
_____

Doctor's Name: _____

Date: _____

Question: _____
_____

Response: _____
_____
_____

Action Plan: _____
_____
_____

Doctor's Name: _____

Date: _____

Question: _____
_____

Response: _____
_____
_____

Action Plan: _____
_____
_____

Lab Tests, X-Rays & Hospital Visits

This section is for keeping track of your family member's lab tests, x-rays or diagnostic tests. Also include any hospitalizations, emergency room, or urgent care visits.

Month: _____ Year: _____

Lab Tests, X-Rays or Hospital Visits/Date	Results	Comments/Follow-Up

Reminders/Shopping List

Date	Things To Do	Shopping List

My Medications

Name Of Drug	Prescribing Doctor And Phone #	Dosage and Frequency	Date You Began Taking It	Date To Stop Taking It	What Condition Does The Drug Treat	Color and Shape	Refill Date	Special Instructions

Date: _____ Daily Log   Day [_____]

Time	Activities/Visitors	Sleep	Caregiver
AM 7:00			
8:00			
9:00			
10:00			
11:00			
PM 12:00			
1:00			
2:00			
3:00			
4:00			
5:00			
6:00			
7:00			
8:00			
9:00			
10:00			
11:00			
AM 12:00			
1:00			
2:00			
3:00			
4:00			
5:00			
6:00			

Care-receiver Questions/Concerns: _____

_____

Day		**Daily Log**

Time	Medications	Food & Beverage
AM 7:00		
8:00		
9:00		
10:00		
11:00		
PM 12:00		
1:00		
2:00		
3:00		
4:00		
5:00		
6:00		
7:00		
8:00		
9:00		
10:00		
11:00		
AM 12:00		
1:00		
2:00		
3:00		
4:00		
5:00		
6:00		

Care-receiver Questions/Concerns: _____

_____

Respite Caregiver Checklist

_____ Generally understands instructions   _____ May not understand instructions

Medical Equipment	When	Needs Assistance	Need to Know
Catheter Care			
Hearing Aid			
Shaving			
Peri-Care			
Mouth/Oral Care			
Bed Sores			
Foley Bag			
Dressings Changed			
Hair/Skin/Nail Care			
Dentures			
Other			

Moving Care-receiver

Moves around unassisted _____   Bedbound _____   Reposition _____   Other _____

Transfers from bed to chair with assistance _____

Walking/Transporting

Unassisted _____   Cane _____   Walker _____   Wheelchair _____

Toileting

Unassisted _____   Bedpan _____   Urinal _____   Catheter _____   Colostomy _____

Bedside Commode _____   Incontinent Pads _____   Other _____

Bathing

Bed Bath _____   Shower _____   Tub _____   Needs Assistance _____ times per week

Equipment Needed:

None _____   Transfer Bench _____   Shower Bench _____   Wheelchair _____

Respite Caregiver Checklist, cont.

Sleeping

Bed Time _____ Wake Time _____ Nap Time(s) _____

Prefers Room Dark _____ Room Temperature _____

Meals/Snacks

Needs assistance feeding _____ Needs to be fed _____ Has difficulty swallowing _____

Takes nothing by mouth _____ Tube feeding _____

Soft foods _____ Record liquid and food intake _____

Avoid _____

House Rules and Instructions

Locked Doors _____

Don't Smoke _____

Oven/Stove Instructions _____

Fireplace _____

Gas/Water Shut Off Valve _____

Fire Extinguishers _____

Visitors _____

Pet Care Guidelines _____

_____

Emergency Preparedness

Discuss 911 preferences _____

Review Emergency Procedures/Info _____

Exit/Escape Plan _____

Advance Directives can be found _____

Other Important Information

_____

_____

_____

_____

End-of-Life Issues Checklist

When planning a funeral, try not to do everything yourself. Call on a family member or friend to help you make the following arrangements.

Funeral/Burial Arrangements

- Know previously made arrangements for cemetery lot, funeral, etc.
- Are wishes known regarding burial/cremation?

A Funeral Checklist

When planning a funeral, try not to do everything yourself. Call on a family member or friend to help you make the following arrangements.

Notify:

- ❏ Doctor
- ❏ Coroner
- ❏ Funeral Home
- ❏ Clergy
- ❏ Relatives and friends
- ❏ Pallbearers
- ❏ Insurance Agents
- ❏ Banks
- ❏ Unions and Fraternal Organizations
- ❏ Organists

Select:

- ❏ Cemetery property
- ❏ Funeral service
- ❏ Casket
- ❏ Vault or outer container
- ❏ Clothing
- ❏ Flowers
- ❏ Music
- ❏ Thank you announcements
- ❏ Transportation
- ❏ Time and place for funeral
- ❏ Time and place for visitation

Provide:

- ❏ Vital statistics about the deceased
- ❏ Birthdate
- ❏ Birthplace
- ❏ Father's name
- ❏ Mother's name
- ❏ Social Security Number
- ❏ Veteran's Discharge or Claim Number
- ❏ Education
- ❏ Marital status

In addition you will want to:

- ❏ Find addresses of all people who must be notified.
- ❏ Make arrangements for out-of-town visitors.
- ❏ Find someone to help answer sympathetic phone calls, cards and letters, as well as greet friends and relatives when they call.
- ❏ Decide appropriate memorial to which gifts may be made (church, hospice, etc.).
- ❏ Prepare list of distant persons to be notified by letter/or printed notice and decide which to send.
- ❏ Locate the will and notify lawyer and executor.
- ❏ Check carefully all life and casualty insurance and death benefits including social security, credit union, fraternal and military.
- ❏ Check promptly on all debts and installment payments, including credit cards. Some carry insurance clauses that cancel balances upon death.
- ❏ Notify utilities and landlord and tell post office where to send mail (if deceased was living alone).

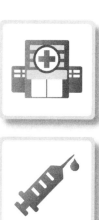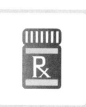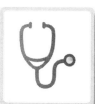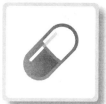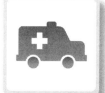

Part 3

Extras

101 Tips

1. First, take good care of yourself.
2. Ask for help. Advocate for what you need.
3. Break the job into small tasks.
4. Give yourself lots of credit.
5. Educate yourself about the care-receiver's condition.
6. Seek support from other caregivers.
7. Plan ahead.
8. Develop a back-up plan.
9. Trust your instincts.
10. Get enough rest and eat properly.
11. Have a sense of humor. Laugh as much as you can.
12. When people offer to help, accept their offer.
13. Get organized.
14. Treat the care-receiver with respect.
15. Forgive yourself for being human.
16. Speak in a simple, clear way.
17. Be aware of other care options and be willing to explore them.
18. Keep supplies together that often used together. Keep a list of supplies so that you can easily replace them.
19. Set aside time for prayer and reflection.
20. Use respite care when needed.
21. Stay in touch with outside friends.
22. Know that you are providing an invaluable and important service to the person you are taking care of.
23. Watch out for signs of depression.
24. Stand up for your rights as a caregiver.
25. Incorporate activities that give your pleasure.
26. Pamper yourself. Listen to music. Get a massage.
27. Try to take a walk everyday.
28. Keep a journal. Write down your thoughts and feelings.
29. Schedule visitors to help give you a break.
30. Join an online support group.
31. Talk to the pharmacist about ways to organize medications.
32. Be realistic in your expectations.
33. Find a support group where you can share your feelings and concerns.
34. Keep in mind that the way the person functions may change from day to day, so try to be flexible and adapt your routine as needed.
35. Avoid talking to the care-receiver like a baby or talking about the person as if he or she weren't there.

101 Tips

36. Minimize distractions and noise—such as the television or radio—to help the person focus on what you are saying.
37. Call the care-receiver by name, making sure you have his or her attention before speaking.
38. Try to frame questions and instructions in a positive way.
39. Plan the bath or shower for the time of day when the care-receiver is most calm and agreeable. Be consistent. Try to develop a routine.
40. Minimize safety risks by using a handheld showerhead, shower bench, grab bars, and nonskid bath mats. Never leave the person alone in the bath or shower.
41. Try to have the care-receiver get dressed at the same time each day so he or she will come to expect it as part of the daily routine.
42. Encourage the person to dress himself or herself to whatever degree possible. Plan to allow extra time so there is no pressure or rush.
43. Aim for a quiet, calm, reassuring mealtime atmosphere by limiting noise and other distractions.
44. Choose dishes and eating tools that promote independence. If the person has trouble using utensils, use a bowl instead of a plate, or offer utensils with large or built-up handles. Use straws or cups with lids to make drinking easier.
45. Help the care-receiver get started on an activity. Break the activity down into small steps and praise the person for each step he or she completes.
46. Have a routine for taking the person to the bathroom and stick to it as closely as possible. For example, take the person to the bathroom every 3 hours or so during the day. Don't wait for the person to ask.
47. Encourage exercise during the day and limit daytime napping, but make sure that the person gets adequate rest during the day because fatigue can increase the likelihood of late afternoon restlessness.
48. Try to keep bedtime at a similar time each evening. Developing a bedtime routine may help.
49. Restrict access to caffeine late in the day.
50. Install secure locks on all outside windows and doors, especially if the person is prone to wandering.
51. Remove the locks on bathroom doors to prevent the person from accidentally locking himself or herself in.
52. Use childproof latches on kitchen cabinets and anyplace where cleaning supplies or other chemicals are kept.
53. Label medications and keep them locked up.
54. Make sure knives, lighters and matches, and guns are secured and out of reach.
55. Keep the house free from clutter.
56. Remove scatter rugs and anything else that might contribute to a fall.
57. Make sure lighting is good both inside and out.
58. Be alert to and address kitchen-safety issues, such as the person forgetting to turn off the stove after cooking. Consider installing an automatic shut-off switch on the stove to prevent burns or fire.
59. Keep or adapt family traditions that are important to you. Include the person with AD as much as possible.
60. Recognize that things will be different, and have realistic expectations about what you can do.
61. Encourage friends and family to visit. Limit the number of visitors at one time, and try to schedule visits during the time of day when the person is at his or her best.
62. Avoid crowds, changes in routine, and strange surroundings that may cause confusion or agitation.

101 Tips

63. Do your best to enjoy yourself.
64. Take time to nurture yourself daily with a healthy diet, exercise and adequate rest and sleep.
65. Organize your responsibilities and priorities.
66. Allow yourself to be angry. Sometimes things do not always go well.
67. Maintain an active social life.
68. Take the time to be with friends.
69. Acknowledge all that you do.
70. Schedule regular afternoons or evenings out.
71. If you can't leave and friends can't come over, take time each day for a phone conversation with a friend or family member.
72. Eat nutritious meals. Don't give in to stress-driven urges for sweets or drink too much alcohol.
73. Get enough sleep. If you are kept up at night, try a nap during the day to make up some sleep.
74. Exercise regularly, even if it means finding someone else to provide care while you walk or go to exercise class.
75. Make a list of jobs you need help with and seek out someone to assist you. This could include household chores, home repair or maintenance, driving, paying bills, or finding information on services you need.
76. If possible, arrange for adult day care for your loved one.
77. Join a support group—online or locally.
78. Draw strength from your faith. Even home visits from a member of your church or synagogue are a way to keep you in touch.
79. Plan a weekend getaway or a week long vacation.
80. Take care of legal matters, both medical and financial.
81. Locate government agencies and learn the procedure to apply for services that can offer financial support (disability), personal care assistants and other supportive services.
82. Understand your medical insurance and the procedure you will have to follow to get assistive devices that are covered by insurance.
83. Get all of your "papers" in one safe place - certified copies of birth certificates, marriage certificate, divorce decree, voter registration, vehicle registration and title, social security card, military identification and discharge orders.
84. You will need legal documents such as a will, power of attorney for healthcare, power of attorney for property, life insurance policies, bank statements, and a listing of all financial accounts.
85. Begin your own medical record (Family Caregiver Organizer) of the care-receiver, including a list of all procedures with dates and all medications (include over the counter.)
86. You should get copies of the medical record whenever you see a specialist or go for a test.
87. Discuss with your care-receiver what issues are more important to him or her, such as staying in his or her own home.
88. Make a list of those you think will be willing to help you and the care-receiver. Make a list of very specific tasks and ask each of them to select what they are willing to do.
89. Keep this list next to the phone, so when someone asks you what they can do, you will have a quick response.
90. Teach others how they can help.
91. Not everything important is urgent.

101 Tips

92. Find balance.
93. Wherever possible, try to make all important decisions **after** a good night's sleep, or a long walk and in the light of day.
94. Never let yourself get too hungry, angry, lonely or tired.
95. Learn to let go.
96. Take care of your back.
97. Focus on the good qualities in a difficult person.
98. Always be direct and to the point.
99. There's a **difference** between caring and doing. Be **open** to technologies and ideas that promote your loved one's independence.
100. Grieve for your losses, and then allow yourself to dream new dreams.
101. Seek **support** from other caregivers. There is great strength in knowing you are not alone.

Resources

AARP
601 E Street, NW
Washington, DC 20049
800-424-3410
Web site: www.aarp.org

Aging with Dignity
PO Box 1661
Tallahassee, FL 32302-1661
888-5-WISHES (594-7437)
Web site:
www.agingwithdignity.org

Alzheimer's Association
800-272-3900
Web site: www.alz.org

American Association of Homes and Services for the Aging
Washington, DC
202-783-2242
Web site: www.AAHSA.org/public

American College of Physicians - American Society of Internal Medicine — ACP-ASIM
Web site: www.acponline.org

American Red Cross
2025 E Street, NW
Washington, DC 20006
202-303-4498
Web site: www.redcross.org

Benefits Check-Up and Benefits Check-Up RX
Web site:
www.benefitscheckup.org

Caregiver Assistance Network (CAN)
100 E. Eighth St.,
Cincinnati, OH 45202
513-241 7745
Web site:
www.cssdoorway.org/can

Children of Aging Parents (CAPS)
1609 Woodbourne Road,
Suite 302A
Levittown, PA 19057
800-227-7294
Web site:
www.caps4caregivers.org

Consumer Consortium on Assisted Living
2342 Oak Street
Falls Church, VA 22046
703-533-8121
Web site: www.ccal.org

Easter Seals
230 West Monroe Street,
Suite 1800
Chicago, IL 60606
800-221-6827
Web site: www.easter-seals.org

National Academy of Elder Law Attorneys, Inc.
1604 North Country Club Rd.
Tucson, Arizona 85716
520-881-4005
Fax 520-325-7925

Eldercare Locator
National Association of Area Agencies on Aging
927 15th Street, NW, 6th floor
Washington, DC 20005
800-677-1116
Web site: www.n4a.org or
www.eldercare.gov

Faith in Action
Wake Forest University School of Medicine
Medical Center Boulevard
Winston-Salem, NC 27157
877-324-8411
Web site: www.fiavolunteers.org

Families USA
Web site: www.familiesusa.org

Family Caregiver Alliance
690 Market Street, Suite 600
San Francisco, CA 94104
415-434-3388
800-445-8106
Web site: www.caregiver.org

**Family Caregivers' Help Center,
The Indiana Association for Home
& Hospice Care, Inc.**
8888 Keystone Crossing,
Suite 1050
Indianapolis, IN 46240
317-844-6630
Web site: www.ind-homecare.org

Resources

Family Friends

National Council on the Aging, Inc.
409 Third Street, SW
Washington, DC 20024
202-479-6672

Family Voices, Inc.

3411 Candelaria NE, Suite M
Albuquerque, NM 87107
888-835-5669
Web site: www.familyvoices.org

Friends' Health Connection

PO Box 114
New Brunswick, NJ 08903
800-483-7436
Web site: www.48friend.org

HealthInsurance.com

800-942-9019
Web site:
www.healthinsurance.com

Hill-Burton Free Medical Care Program

800-638-0742
Web site: www.hrsa.gov/osp/dfcr

Home Care Companions

1320 Divisadero St.,
San Francisco, CA 94115
415-824-3269
Web site:
www.homecarecompanions.org

Hospice Foundation of America

2001 S Street, NW, Suite 300
Washington, DC 20009
800-854-3402
Web site:
www.hospicefoundation.org

Last Acts

Web site: www.lastacts.org

Me and My Caregiver(s)

PO Box 157
Chelsea, MI 48118
734-458-1098
Web site:
www.MeAndMyCaregivers.com

Medicare Rights Center

1460 Broadway, 11th Floor
New York, NY 10036
888-HMO-9050
Web site:
www.medicarerights.org

Medicine Program

PO Box 515
Doniphan, MO 63935
573-996-7300
Web site:
www.themedicineprogram.com

National Adult Day Services Association, Inc.

8201 Greensboro Drive, Suite 300
McLean, VA 22102
866-890-7357
Web site: www.nadsa.org

National Alliance for Caregiving

4720 Montgomery Lane, 5th Floor
Bethesda, MD 20814
Web site: www.caregiving.org

National Association for Home Care and Hospice

228 7th Street, SE
Washington, DC 20003
202-547-7424
Web site: www.nahc.org

National Association of Hospital Hospitality Houses (NAHHH)

P.O. Box 18087
Asheville, NC 28814
800-542-9730
Web site: www.nahhh.org

National Caregiving Foundation

801 N. Pitt St., #116,
Alexandria, VA 22314-1765
703-299-9300

National Citizens' Coalition for Nursing Home Reform

1424 16th Street, NW, Suite 202
Washington, DC 20036
202-332-2275
Web site: www.nccnhr.org

National Family Caregivers Association

10400 Connecticut Avenue, Ste 500
Kensington, MD 20895
800-896-3650
Web site:
www.thefamilycaregiver.org

National Hospice and Palliative Care Organization

1700 Diagonal Road, Suite 625
Alexandria, VA 22314
800-658-8898
Web site: www.nhpco.org

National Patient Travel Center

Mercy Medical Airlift
4620 Haygood Road, Suite 1
Virginia Beach, VA 23455
800-296-1217
Web site: www.PatientTravel.org

Resources

National Respite Coalition
4016 Oxford Street
Annandale, VA 22003
703-256-9578
Web site:
www.archrespite.org/NRC.htm

National Respite Locator Service
800 Eastowne Drive, Suite 105
Chapel Hill, NC 27514
800-473-1727, ext. 222
Web site: www.respitelocator.org

New LifeStyles
4144 N. Central Expressway, Suite 1000
Dallas, TX 75204
800-869-9549
Web site: www.newlifestyles.com

Partnership for Caring: America's Voice for the Dying
Web site:
www.partnershipforcaring.org

Patient Advocate Foundation
700 Thimble Shoals Boulevard, Suite 200
Newport News, VA 23606
800-532-5274
Web site:
www.patientadvocate.org

Rosalynn Carter Institute for Human Development
800 Wheatley Street
Americus, GA 31709
229-928-1234
Web site: www.rci.gsw.edu

Shepherd's Centers of America
One West Armour Boulevard, Suite 201
Kansas City, MO 64111
800-547-7073
Web site:
www.shepherdcenters.org

Supportive Care of the Dying
c/o Providence Health System
4805 NE Glisan Street, 2E07
Portland, Oregon 97213
tel: (503- 215-5053
fax: (503- 215-5054
Web site: www.careofdying.org

The Center for Family Caregivers
P.O. Box 224
Park Ridge IL 60068
847-823-0639
Web site:
www.Familycaregivers.org

The Compassionate Friends
P.O. Box 3696
Oak Brook, IL 60522
877-969-0010
Web site:
www.compassionatefriends.org

The National Association of Professional Geriatric Care Managers
1604 North Country Club Road
Tucson, AZ 85716
520-881-8008
Web site: www.caremanager.org

U.S. Administration on Aging
Department of Health and Human Services
Washington, DC 20201
202-619-0724
Web site: www.aoa.gov

Visiting Nurse Associations of America
617-737-3200
Web site: www.vnaa.org

Well Spouse Foundation
63 West Main Street, Suite H
Freehold, NJ 07728
800-838-0879
Web site: www.wellspouse.org

Glossary

Accelerated Death Benefit

A life insurance policy benefit that lets the insured person use some of the policy's death benefit prior to death for purposes such as long-term care.

Activities of Daily Living (ADLs)

Basic personal activities, which include bathing, eating, dressing, mobility, transferring from bed to chair, and using the toilet. ADLs are used to measure how dependent a person may be on assistance in performing any or all of these activities.

Acute Care

The care provided for a medical condition from which a patient is expected to recover and resume a "normal" lifestyle, even though it may not be the same as before onset of the condition. Acute care usually refers to physician and/or hospital services of less than three months' duration.

Acute Pain

Pain that has a known cause and occurs for a limited time.

Administration on Aging (AOA)

An agency of the US Department of Health and Human Services.

Adult Care Home

Also called board and care home or group home, an adult care home is a residence that offers housing and personal care services, such as meals, supervision, and transportation for 3 to 16 residents.

Adult Day Care

Community-based care designed to meet the needs of functionally and/or cognitively impaired adults who, for their own safety and well-being, can no longer be left at home alone during the day.
Adult day centers offer protected settings which are normally open five days a week during business hours and include a mixture of health, social an support services. Many programs provide meals and transportation services to and from a patients home, and specialized programs for individuals with Alzheimer's disease or related disorders. These programs often provide a respite, or break for family caregivers.

Adult Guardian

The person appointed by a court, usually a probate or surrogate court, to perform court-ordered tasks of caring for an incapacitated adult's financial affairs and personal needs.

Adult Protective Services

State or county run program(s) designed to protect adults who may be physically, emotionally or financially abused and/or neglected.

Advance Directive for Health Care

A written document that specifies how the signer wants medical decisions to be made. A health care advance directive may include a Living Will, a Durable Power of Attorney for Health Care or both.

Allied Health Professionals

Persons with special training in fields related to medicine, such as medical social work and physical or occupational therapy. Allied health professionals work with physicians or other health professionals.

Alzheimer's Disease

A progressive, neurodegenerative disease characterized by loss of function and death of nerve sells in several areas of the brain, leading to loss of mental functions such as memory and learning. Alzheimer's disease is the most common cause of dementia.

Ambulatory Aids

Ambulatory aids include a range of devices to help seniors move about safely and independently when additional support is needed. Types of ambulatory aids include: walkers, cruisers, forearm crutches, canes, wheelchairs, and motorized scooters. These aids are often paid for by Medicare/Medicaid or private insurance.

Ambulatory Care

All types of health services that are provided on an outpatient basis, instead of services provided in the home or to persons in a clinical setting.

Ambulatory with Assistance

Able to get about with the aid of a cane, crutch, brace, wheelchair or walker.

Glossary

Ambulatory

Able to walk about.

Ancillary Services

Those services needed by a nursing home resident, but not provided by a nursing home, such as podiatry, dentistry, etc., and which may not be included in the basic rate of the facility.

Annuity

A series of payments made periodically for a specific period of time. The payment amounts can be variable or fixed. Many insurance companies sell a wide variety of annuity contracts with payments that begin immediately upon purchase of the contract or are deferred until some time in the future. Some annuity contracts waive their surrender charges (early withdrawal penalties) in the event of a lengthy hospital stay, nursing home confinement, or terminal illness.

Area Agency on Aging (AAA)

Local government agency that grants or contracts with public and private organizations to provide services for older persons, created by a provision of The Older Americans Act. Services include information and referral for in-home services, counseling, legal services, adult day care, skilled nursing care/therapy, transportation, personal care, respite care, nutrition and meals.

Assessment

Activities performed by at least one professional (preferably a social worker and/or a nurse) to determine a person's current ability to function in six areas: physical health, mental health, social support, activities of daily living, environmental conditions, and financial situation.

Assignment

A method of billing Medicare for services. The provider agrees to bill Medicare directly for services and agrees to accept Medicare's allowed charge as payment in full. Medicare pays the provider directly. The provider can then bill the beneficiary for deductibles and coinsurance.

Assisted Living Facility (ALF)

Residences that provide a "home with services" and that emphasize residents' privacy and choice. Assisted living residence means any group housing and services program for two or more unrelated adults, that makes available, at a minimum, one meal a day and housekeeping services and provides personal care services to the residents. Settings in which services are delivered may include self-contained apartment units or single or shared room units with private or area baths.

Assistive Devices

A range of products designed to help seniors or people with disabilities lead more independent lives. Examples include motorized wheelchairs, walking aids, elevated toilet seats, bathtub seats, and handrails.

Attorney-in-Fact

In legal terms, the person who is granted power-of-attorney.

Benefit Maximum

The limit a health insurance policy will pay for a certain loss or covered service. The benefit can be expressed either as 1) a length of time (e.g., 60 days), or 2) a dollar amount (e.g., $350 for a specific illness or procedure), or 3) a percentage of the Medicare approved amount. The benefits may be paid to the policyholder or to a third party. This may refer to a specific illness, time frame or the life of the policy.

Benefit Period

The number of years an insurance policy will provide benefits. Many long-term care insurance policies offer terms between three and five years. Some offer lifetime benefits.

Bereavement

The act of grieving someone's death.

Burnout

The feeling of becoming overly frustrated and negative experienced by some caregivers.

Care Manager

A health care professional, typically a nurse or social worker, who arranges, monitors or coordinates long-term care services. Also referred to as a care coordinator or case manager.

Glossary

Care Plan

A written action plan that contains the strategies for delivering care to address an individual's needs and problems.

Care-Receiver

The person receiving care.

Caregiver

An adult who provides unpaid care for the physical and emotional needs of a family member or friend.

Certified Nursing Assistant (CNA)

CNAs are trained and certified to help nurses by providing non-medical assistance to patients, such as help with eating, cleaning and dressing.

Certified

A long-term care facility, home health agency, or hospice agency that meets the requirements imposed by Medicare and Medicaid is said to be certified. Being certified is not the same as being accredited. Medicare, Medicaid and some long-term care insurance policies only cover care in a certified facility or provided by a certified agency.

Chair Bound

Unable to get out of a chair without the help of another person.

Chronic Illness

A physical or mental disability that continues or recurs frequently over a long period of time; often associated with disability.

Chronic Pain

Pain that occurs for more than one month after healing of an injury, that occurs repeatedly over months, or that is due to a lesion that is not expected to heal.

Co-Existing Illness

A medical condition or illness that occurs simultaneously with another and may complicate or obscure diagnosis or treatment of each.

Companion Services

Volunteers, business and agencies that provide friendly assistance and companionship to elders. Can include conversation, light housekeeping and meal preparation, running errands and providing transportation.

Competence

Usually used in a legal sense, refers to a person's ability to understand information, make an informed choice based on the information and values, and communicate that decision.

Comprehensive

A full range of available services including various levels of nursing care, support therapies, psycho/social assessments, treatment and referral to appropriate resources.

Conservator

Person appointed by the court in a legal proceeding to act as the legal representative of a person who is mentally or physically incapable of managing his or her own affairs.

Continence

The ability to maintain control of bowel and bladder function. Or, when unable to maintain control of these functions, the ability to perform associated personal hygiene (including caring for catheter or colostomy bag).

Continuing Care Retirement Community (CCRC)

A retirement community that offers a broad range of services and levels of care based on what each resident needs over time. Sometimes called "life care," it can range from independent living in an apartment to assisted living to full-time care in a nursing home.

CPR

Cardio-Pulmonary Resuscitation.

Custodial Care

Care to help individuals meet personal needs such as bathing, dressing, eating, and other non-medical care that most people do themselves, such as using eye drops. Medicare does not pay for custodial care and Medicaid pays very little.

Dehydration

Lack of adequate fluid in the body and a crucial factor in the health of older people.

Glossary

Dementia

The loss of intellectual functions such as thinking, remembering and reasoning to the extent that a person's daily functioning is affected. It is not a disease in itself, but rather a group of symptoms which may accompany certain diseases or physical conditions. The cause and rate of progression of dementia vary.

Discharge Planner

A social worker or other health care professional who assists hospital patients and their families in transitioning from the hospital to another level of care such as rehabilitation in a skilled nursing facility, home health care in the patient's home, or long-term care in a nursing home.

Do Not Resuscitate Order (DNR)

A code or order indicating that in the event a patient's heart or breathing stops, there should be no intervention. This does not mean that the individual does not receive care. Continuing care is provided as it would to any individual (medications for pain, antibiotics, etc.) except as stated above.

Durable Medical Equipment

Medical equipment that is ordered by a doctor for use in the home. These items, such as walkers, wheelchairs, and hospital beds, must be reusable. Durable medical equipment is paid for under Medicare, subject to a 20% coinsurance of the Medicare-approved amount.

Durable Power of Attorney for Health Care (DPOAHC)

A legal document that specifies one or more individuals (called a health care proxy) designated to make medical decisions for a person if that person is incapacitated.

Elder Law Attorney

An attorney who specializes in the laws that deal with the rights and issues of the health, finances, and well-being of the elderly and the power of other individuals and the government to control them.

Eldercare

A wide range of services provided at home, in the community and in residential care facilities, including assisted living facilities and nursing homes. It includes health-related services such as rehabilitative therapies, skilled nursing, and palliative care, as well as supervision and a wide range of supportive personal care and social services.

Executor

The person or institution appointed in a will, or by a court, to settle the estate of a deceased person.

Family Caregiver

Anyone who provides care without pay and who usually has personal ties to the care recipient. This person can provide full or part time help, and may live with the care recipient or separately.

Gatekeeper

A term sometimes used to refer to HMO primary care physicians or nurse practitioners because of their responsibility for referring members to specialists or other services.

Geriatric Care Manager

One who develops and implements a plan for all aspects of long-term care to assist an elderly person and, indirectly, the person's family members.
A geriatric care manager will usually hold a graduate degree, and may be certified or licensed by a professional organization or by state statute or regulations.

Geriatrician

A medical doctor with special education and training in the diagnosis, treatment, and prevention of disabilities in older people.

Gerontologist

A professional who specializes in the mental and behavioral characteristics of aging.

Guardian

An individual appointed by a court of law to manage a person's financial and/or personal affairs because the court has found that the person is not competent to manage his or her own affairs. A conservator is similarly appointed, but only for financial affairs.

Home Health Agency

An organization that provides home care services, including skilled nursing care, physical therapy, occu-

Glossary

pational therapy, speech therapy, and care by home health aides.

Home Health Aide

A person who provides personal care including bathing, dressing and grooming, and some household services.

Home Health Care

Health services provided in the homes of the elderly, disabled, sick, or convalescent. The types of services provided include nursing care, social services, home health aide and homemaking services, and various rehabilitation therapies (e.g., speech, physical and occupational therapy).

Hospice

Medical and social programs for terminally ill patients and families either at home or in a facility. Hospice care emphasizes pain control, symptom management, and emotional support rather than life-sustaining equipment.

Incompetence

A legal determination that one is incapable of handling assets and exercising certain legal rights.

Incontinence

The loss of bowel and bladder control.

Instrumental Activities of Daily Living (IADLs)

Personal tasks often performed by a caregiver, such as meal preparation, grocery shopping, making telephone calls, and money management.

Intermittent Care

Skilled nursing and home health aide services furnished up to 28 hours per week over any number of days per week so long as they are offered less than 8 hours per day.

Licensed Practical Nurse (LPN)

One who has completed one or two years in a school of nursing or vocational training school. LPNs are in charge of nursing in the absence of a Registered Nurse (RN). LPNs often give medications and perform treatments. They are licensed by the state in which they work.

Living Will

A document that makes known a person's wishes regarding medical treatments in the event the person becomes incompetent or is unable to speak.

Long-Term Care

A general term that describes a range of medical, nursing, custodial, social, and community services designed to help people with chronic health impairments or forms of dementia.

Long-Term Care Facilities

Institutions that provide nursing care to people who are unable to care for themselves and who may have health problems ranging from minimal to serious. These facilities are often used for short-term rehabilitation after hospitalization.

Long-Term Care Insurance

This type of insurance policy is designed to cover long term care expenses in a facility or at home. Neither Medicare nor Medicare supplemental insurance (Medigap) will pay for these expenses.

Long-Term Care Ombudsman Programs

Independent, nationwide, federally-funded services that work to resolve problems between residents and assisted living facilities, nursing homes and other residential care facilities.

Medicaid

An assistance program through which the federal government and the individual states share in payment for the medical care of certain categories of needy and low-income people.

Medicare

A federal health insurance program for people 65 and over and some under 65 who are disabled. Medicare has two parts. Part A is also called Hospital Insurance, and Part B is called Medical Insurance.

Medicare Supplemental Insurance (Medigap)

This is private insurance (often called Medigap) that pays Medicare's deductibles and co-insurances, and may cover services not covered by Medicare. Most Medigap plans will help pay for skilled nursing care, but only when that care is covered by Medicare.

Glossary

Nursing Home

An institutional setting that offers 24-hour supervision and care to individuals, usually older persons, who are no longer able to be responsible for themselves in an independent living setting.

Nutrition/Hydration (IV)

Intravenous (IV) fluid and nutritional supplements given to patients who are unable to eat or drink by mouth, or those who are dehydrated or malnourished.

Palliative Care

The total care of patients with progressive, incurable illness. In palliative care, the focus of care is on quality of life. Control of pain and other physical symptoms, and psychological, social and spiritual problems are considered most important.

Power of Attorney

The simplest and least expensive legal device for authorizing a person to manage the affairs of another.

PRN

An abbreviation used to indicate that a medication is given or treatment performed only as the need arises.

Registered Nurse (RN)

A graduate nurse who has completed a minimum of two years of education at an accredited school of nursing. RNs are licensed by the state in which they work.

Residential Care Facility

A generic term for a group home, specialized apartment complex or other institution that provides care services where individuals live. The term is used to refer to a range of residential care options including assisted living facilities, board and care homes and skilled nursing facilities.

Respite Care

Temporary caregiving services provided when the primary caretaker needs time away from caregiving. Respite care is provided in-home or an alternative location for a short stay.

Self Care

The ability to bathe, dress, toilet, and feed oneself.

Senior Group Home

Senior group homes are small, private homes, often located in residential neighborhoods that provide assisted living services for a small number of seniors who live together. Residents share in the daily living responsibilities and support services provided by at least on supervisor who usually lives on-site. Senior group home residents typically require limited medical care, but meals, housekeeping, and personal care services may be provided. Residents benefit from the close-knit community atmosphere of this long-term living arrangement.

Skilled Care

Institutional care that is less intensive than hospital care in its nursing and medical service, but which includes procedures that require the training and skills of an RN for administration. Both Medicare and Medicaid reimburse for care at the skilled level if it is provided in a facility that has been certified as meeting the Skilled Nursing Facility (SNF) standards.

Skilled Nursing Facility (SNF)

A facility that has been certified by Medicare and/or Medicaid to provide skilled care.

Spend Down

Under the Medicaid program, a method by which an individual establishes Medicaid eligibility by reducing gross income through incurring medical expenses until net income (after medical expenses) meets Medicaid financial requirements. A resident spends down when he/she is no longer sufficiently covered by a third-party payor (usually Medicare) and has exhausted all personal assets. The resident then becomes eligible for Medicaid coverage.

Veterans Administration (VA)

The Department of Military and Veterans Affairs administers a variety of programs to assist veterans and their families.

Vital Signs

Temperature, pulse, respiration, and blood pressure.

Alzheimer's Disease and Caregiving

What is Alzheimer's disease?

Alzheimer's disease is the most common form of dementia. More than five million Americans now have Alzheimer's. People with Alzheimer's disease have abnormal amyloid plaques and neurofibrillary tangles. As the disease progresses, symptoms include confusion, trouble with organizing and expressing thoughts, misplacing things, getting lost in familiar places, and changes in personality and behavior.

What is the difference between dementia and Alzheimer's disease?

Dementia is not a disease. It is a group of symptoms that may result from certain diseases or physical disorders. Alzheimer's disease is the most common form of dementing diseases. It is a progressive, degenerative disease that attacks the brain and results in impaired memory, thinking, and behavior.

What are the stages of Alzheimer's disease?

It is often difficult to determine which stage a patient is in because they frequently overlap.

The stages include:

- No impairment-no symptoms.
- Very mild decline. Mild forgetfulness, vague about familiar things, forgets well known names.
- Mild decline. Mild confusion, gets lost going to familiar places, loses things, has trouble concentrating.
- Moderate decline (mild or early stage). Cannot handle money, avoids complex tasks, withdraws from challenging situations.
- Moderately severe decline (moderate or mid-stage). Dementia sets in, needs assistance in grooming, confused about times and dates.
- Severe decline (moderately severe or mid-stage). Severe decline, forgets name of spouse, entirely dependent, trouble with normal sleep pattern.
- Very severe decline (severe or late stage). Verbal abilities lost, needs help eating and going to the bathroom, loses ability to walk.

How long can a person live with Alzheimer's disease?

The progression of the disease varies from person to person. On average, Alzheimer's patients live from eight to ten years after they are diagnosed. On average, the early stages may last two to four years, the middle stages from two to ten years, and the last stages from about one to three years.

What are some of the biggest challenges that Alzheimer's caregivers face?

Alzheimer's caregivers have to deal with the difficult behaviors of the care-receivers. Dressing, bathing, and eating often become difficult to manage. Each day brings new challenges as the care-receiver's disease progresses. The care-receiver cannot be left unattended, even for a few minutes at a time. Caring for a person with Alzheimer's can be overwhelming. It is important to have a care plan and a good support system.

What are the top 10 caregiving tips for Alzheimer's caregivers?

1. Educate yourself about Alzheimer's disease.
2. Ask the doctor any questions you may have about the disease. Be alert to changes in the care-receiver.
3. Find an Alzheimer's disease support group.
4. Develop a care plan. Keep in mind that the way the care-receiver functions may change from day to day. Try to be flexible and adaptable.
5. Make the environment soothing, familiar and calming. Avoid too much stimulation. Use familiar routines.
6. Keep the home safe. You may have to put locks on closets, gate guards, etc.
7. Stay calm. The Alzheimer patient may often mimic the caregiver's emotions.
8. Adjust your expectations. Accept and validate the care-receiver's view of reality. Remember, people with Alzheimer's disease may see the world in different, amusing, or disorganized ways. Allow their reality to exist.
9. Expect some behavioral problems. A person with Alzheimer's disease has limited ability to learn and adapt. He/she often reacts to any stress or demands by displaying agitation or disruptive behavior. Don't take it personally. Realize that the disease is responsible for the behavior.

Consider using adult day care or respite services to ease the day-to-day demands of caregiving.

Bonus: Caring for the Caregiver

Caring for someone who is chronically ill, or who requires constant attention, is an extremely demanding job. Caregivers owe it to themselves to recognize and care for their own needs, in addition to those of the patient. In a perfect world, the care-receiver would recognize this and try to minimize the negative effects on their caregiver. As we all know, this is not a perfect world.

Keep in mind that what may be extremely stressful for you, may be a minor irritation for someone else, and maybe not at all stressful to a third person. It is mainly your perception, interpretation, and response to an event. However, certain events (such as long term caregiving) tend to be viewed as highly stressful by most people, most of the time.

Stress can make you sick — physically, emotionally, or both at the same time. Take responsibility for your personal well being and getting your own needs met. Sometimes this is easier said than done. Sometimes, good caregiving can be overwhelming if you do not take steps to keep yourself in good shape.

Understanding And Identifying The Effects of Stress

Stress is the "wear and tear" our bodies experience as we adjust to our constantly changing environment. The stress response is a natural chemical reaction that is intended to help us adequately react to extreme situations. It has both physical and emotional effects on us and can create both positive and negative feelings. However, chronic stress (when the stress demand doesn't go away and the stress hormones don't turn off) wears down the body systems.

When you are under stress, your muscles contract. All of us have experienced tight neck muscles or a clenched jaw at some point in our lives. For most people, these physical symptoms of stress alleviate themselves over time. Being a caregiver might not allow you to dissipate the stress. Muscle tension can affect your nerves, blood vessels, organs, skin, and bones. Over time, chronically tense muscles can lead to a variety of ailments.

Psychologist Dr. Albert Ellis explains the ABC Model of Stress:

A is the **A**ctivating event or potentially stressful situation.

B is your **B**eliefs, thoughts or perceptions about A.

C is the emotional **C**onsequence or stress that results from holding these beliefs.

Good stress can help compel us to action. It can result in a new awareness and an exciting new perspective. However, bad stress can result in feelings of anger, rejection, distrust, and depression. Stress is a part of everyday life. We cannot eliminate it, but we can learn ways to manage it.

Caregiver stress is the emotional strain of caregiving. Full-time caregiving for a chronically ill person can provoke surprising feelings that can lead to physical and/or emotional problems. It is important that we take care of ourselves as we care for our loved one. Watch for the signs and symptoms of stress that our bodies may be sending. You need to self-evaluate every day as long as you are a caregiver.

Do you have any of the common signs of stress? Just how stressed are you? Put a check mark by any symptoms you may be having.

Physical Symptoms

_____ Blurred vision

_____ Muscle tension; pain in the shoulders, back, neck, jaw, knot in stomach

_____ Constricted throat

_____ Headaches

_____ Dilated pupils

_____ Chest pains

_____ Rashes, hives, ulcers

_____ Difficulty in breathing, shortness of breath

_____ Cold, sweaty hands and feet

_____ Spastic colon

_____ Elevated cholesterol

_____ Increased blood pressure

_____ Increased heart rate, rapid pulse

_____ Increased overall metabolic rate

_____ Sleep disorders
_____ Digestive problems
_____ TMJ

Behavioral Symptoms

_____ Always in a hurry
_____ Frequently tardy or absent
_____ Loss of efficiency
_____ Inability to concentrate
_____ Lack of motivation
_____ Fault finding
_____ Verbal or physical abuse
_____ Angry outbursts
_____ Crying or yelling
_____ Nagging or complaining
_____ Inability to relax or enjoy yourself
_____ Depressed
_____ Loss of appetite
_____ Sexual problems
_____ Frequent mood shifts
_____ Withdrawn

Intellectual/Emotional Symptoms

_____ Loss of self-esteem
_____ Loss of healthy attitude on life
_____ Frustration and anger
_____ Depression and pessimism
_____ Life losing its meaning
_____ Inability to concentrate
_____ Forgetfulness
_____ Loss of sense of humor
_____ Inability to enjoy life's pleasures
_____ Loneliness
_____ Internalizing
_____ Guilt and shame

Escape Activities

_____ Smoking
_____ Alcohol and/or drug use
_____ Overeating
_____ Compulsive gambling
_____ Compulsive shopping

More About Stress

To better manage stress it may be necessary to modify the source of stress and/or change your reaction to it. Focus on these eight steps:

1. Become aware of your stressors and your reactions. Don't gloss over your problems.
2. Recognize what you can change and change what you can.
3. Reduce the intensity of your emotional reactions to stress. Are your expectations accurate?
4. Learn to moderate your physical reactions to stress. Take deep, slow breaths.
5. Build your physical reserves. Exercise.
6. Maintain your emotional reserves. Be kind to yourself.
7. Find someone you can talk to about what you are feeling. Join a support group.
8. If you cannot change the situation and cannot change the way you view the situation, you can still manage stress by mastering other skills. You can learn to "turn off" your stress.

Remember, unchecked stress is the number one cause of "caregiver burnout." It is important that you take good care of yourself. In the process you will become a better caregiver.

Schedule regular respite breaks.

Be proactive. You should make an exercise plan, both physical and mental, and stick to it so that you are ready to handle stressful situations, when they arise.

Stress And Your Health

Take the following steps to make your health a priority:

- See your doctor for a checkup.
- Diet. Maintain good nutrition. Eat a diet rich in fruits, vegetables, and whole grains and low saturated fats. Drink plenty of water or other nutritious beverages. Limit or avoid excess salt, alcohol, nicotine and caffeine.
- Rest. Get adequate rest and sleep. Take naps when you can.
- Exercise. Physical and mental exercises are essential tools in keeping the body healthy and functional. Find time to exercise every day.
- Meditation and relaxation. Practice deep breathing and stretching techniques.
- Ask for and accept help from others.
- Get away from it all. Schedule regular respite breaks.
- Let off steam. Find an activity (walking or jogging) to help vent feelings of anger and frustration.
- Stay in touch with friends and family. Social activities can help you feel connected. Loneliness is a major cause of stress.
- Develop a sense of humor. Learn to laugh. Laughter is good for the soul.
- Share the work load. Build a network of people who can help with various tasks. Never attempt to "go it alone".
- Prioritize. Make lists and establish a daily routine. Recognize that you may not accomplish everything on a list, every day. Reset your priorities for the next day.
- Take advice and criticism with a grain of salt. Unless they have been caregivers themselves, they are unable to understand your unique set of problems.
- Take one day at a time and enjoy life whenever possible.

Stress And Your Feelings

Caregivers are often surprised at some of the feelings they have. If any of those feelings are judged as unacceptable, there may be an unconscious tendency to try and hide them. If they are masked or hidden they are major contributors to stress.

How can that be? We can choose our own feelings and behavior. Feelings are created by the way we perceive a situation. Recognize that feelings are neither good or bad. Recognize that while all feelings are okay, all actions are not.

A feeling is defined as an emotional response or an affective state of consciousness, such as that resulting from emotions, sentiments, or desires, to things going on around us.

It is important to know that by changing our thoughts, we can change the way we feel and respond to a situation. We can learn to modify our feelings since they are a by-product of thoughts and messages we send to ourselves. Often this is easier said that done. It takes some practice to make changes. To see changes you have to make changes.

Over time we develop defenses for personal survival. These defenses usually operate on an unconscious level. It is important to make sure you do not bury your pain. Explore your feelings and defenses. Ask yourself these questions:

- What messages is my body sending me right now about my feelings? Stop and identify and acknowledge your personal defenses.
- What defenses am I using to disguise my feelings? Recognize how these are used to bury painful or unpleasant feelings.
- If I ignore these defenses, what feelings come to the surface?
- What caregiving activities trigger these feelings?
- Who can I share these feelings with? Sharing feelings with someone you trust is a healthy way to deal with emotional stress.

Stress Management And Relief

Just as there are many sources of stress, there are many possibilities for its management.

Basically you have to figure out what you are doing that is contributing to your stress and change it.

These changes fall into four categories:

- change your behavior
- change your thinking
- change your lifestyle choices, and/or
- change the situations you are in

By getting to the root causes of your stress, you can relieve current problems and symptoms and you can also prevent recurrences.

A common source of stress is unrealistic expectations. People often become upset about something, not because it is innately stressful, but because it does not concur with what they expected.

Another common source of stress may be because of your belief system.

It is important to articulate your beliefs and then to label them as such. Next, you need to acknowledge that your assumptions are not truth but rather opinions and, therefore, they can be challenged. Lastly, you need to admit that the beliefs held by the other person may be just as valid as your own.

Another form of stress relief is through ventilation – venting or sharing our feelings with a friend. Many caregivers find it helpful to keep a stress journal.

A daily journal will help you focus your efforts and act as a reminder that your stress needs tending to!

Sample Stress Journal

Date: _____ Time: _____

Stressful event: _____
_____
_____

Signs of stress/physical response: _____
_____
_____

Thoughts and feelings experienced with stressful event: _____
_____
_____

What I did that caused symptoms to go away: _____
_____
_____

Comments on this experience: _____
_____
_____

Laughter for Relieving Stress

Laughter reduces the level of stress hormones. Laughter provides a physical and emotional release. Laughter brings the focus away from anger, guilt, stress and negative emotions in a more complete way than mere distractions.

In order to laugh sincerely, you have to let go. Practice laughing. Allow yourself to experience your natural humor. Do not take yourself too seriously. You will find it is difficult to remain tense while laughing.

Watch some funny movies with the care-receiver. They will be good for both of you. So smile more, and laugh even if you do not feel like it. You will still achieve positive effects, and you may be surprised that real smiles, genuine laughter and merriment will follow.

Exercise for Relieving Stress

Physical exercise is one of the most effective ways of relieving stress. Getting into better shape improves your mental health as well as your physical health. Even if you can only exercise ten minutes at a time, it is good for you.

Mark down exercise time in your calendar on a daily basis. Make your best guess as to when you will have time available and if events get in the way, slide the time, do not cancel your exercise period.

Breathing Exercises for Relieving Stress

When you are facing a stressful situation, you can reduce stress by deep breathing. Try this: Sit comfortably with your back straight. Put one hand on your chest and the other on your stomach. Inhale through your nose and the hand on your stomach should begin to rise. Your other hand should move very little. Exhale as much air as you can while contracting your stomach muscles. Once again, the hand on your stomach should move in as you exhale.

Mediation for Relieving Stress

When you meditate you bring together all of the mind's energies and focus them on a word, a sound, a symbol, a comforting image, or your own breathing.

For a simple mediation, try this:

Sit with your back straight and legs comfortably crossed. Try to keep your attention on your breathing and on sensations arising from your body, for fifteen or twenty minutes.

You can learn basic meditation from books or attend classes or retreats for more intensive training. You should practice meditation on a daily basis. Remember, we want to be proactive about combatting stress. Daily meditations will prepare you to handle stress better.

Guided Imagery or Visualization

If you use this method, you will imagine a scene in which you feel at peace, able to let go of all concerns and tensions.

In guided imagery, audio instructions help you visualize the scene, focus your thoughts and relax.

For example, you may listen to a CD that has soft music playing in the background while some one says the following:

Let your thoughts settle and your mind become like a clear lake. Experience the feeling of emptiness. There is no internal dialogue between the various aspects of yourself, just complete calm. As you rest in emptiness, allow your intuition to send you important messages. Sense each message with your mind like a wave rolling up on a clear beach.

Experience a hollow bamboo flute in the center of your upper torso aligned from your head to pelvic floor. Let all of the excess tension locked in your head and shoulders drain down the hollow tube to settle in your one point, located approximately one inch below your navel.

Feel your energy congregating in your one point as your body becomes powerful. You are now immovable and unliftable. Begin walking, you have stability and balance.

Practice placing your attention on the one point during your daily caregiving activities, then you will begin experiencing emptiness.

Yoga for Relieving Stress

Yoga is a broad term for a series of personal practices, which bring together your physical, mental and spiritual resources with the goal of attaining a state of wholeness and completeness.

Hatha yoga teaches you a series of stationary and moving poses called asanas and a form of breath control called pranayama, as well as concentration techniques.

Yoga postures are designed to balance the different systems of the body, including the central nervous, the endocrine and digestive systems. By slowing down your mental activity, taking your mind off the causes of stress, and having gently stretched your body in ways that massage your internal organs; yoga helps you to create dynamic peacefulness within yourself.

Other Ways to Relieve Stress

Try some of these to help relax:

- Listen to soothing music.
- Take a long hot bath or shower.
- Look at a beautiful scene or picture.
- Use aromatherapy, or various scents, to evoke physical responses.
- Chat with a good friend.

Practice taking good care of yourself. Practice these five steps:

1. Forgive yourself — with no strings attached.
2. Forgive others.
3. Don't compare yourself with others.
4. See your good side — don't dwell on the bad.
5. Exchange weak thoughts with strong thoughts.

- Make a list of YOUR warning signs of stress.
- Next, identify the cause of stress in order to find solutions.

Symptoms	Cause	Solution

Of the causes you have listed, which creates the most stress for you?

- Write down every solution you can think of that may reduce or eliminate stress.
- Using your solutions' list, create an action plan to reduce stress. Creating an action plan doesn't have to be complicated.

1. Stress Symptom(s): _____
   _____
   Caused by what event(s): _____
   _____
   Can I alter the event: _____
   _____

2. Activity to reduce stress symptoms:
   Physical activity: _____
   _____
   Mental activity: _____
   _____

3. Schedule for stress reducing activity
   _____ In response to an event
   _____ Daily maintenance prior to an event

4. To get started with a new activity, I will:
   _____
   _____
   _____
   _____
   _____
   _____
   _____
   _____

Conclusion

It really is a wonderful thing, taking care of a loved one in their times of need. Many people make sacrifices in their own lives in order to take care of others. However, all too often the caregiver ignores their own health needs. That can have disastrous consequences not only for the caregiver, but the care-receiver as well. Daily attention is needed for your good physical and mental well-being.

We hope you will create your own daily regimen that will help maintain your health, make you a better caregiver and, therefore, allow you to take better care of your loved one. And you will enjoy the caregiving experience more, if you are in good health.

www.MeAndMyCaregivers.com

Store your caregiving records online

Please visit our web site and bookmark it as a valuable caregiving resource. In addition to caregiving tips and resources, we also offer an electronic organizer of caregiving records. This powerful communications tool will help to promote a dialog between the care-receiver, caregivers, family members and health care providers; and to enhance their ability to provide the best care.

The online organizer provides a step-by-step, systematic approach for recording and storing essential daily records, designed to improve care-receiver satisfaction while enhancing the quality of their health care.

www.MeAndMyCaregivers.com is the first ever online storage site for caregiving records. This subscription site is a critical component of health care. It enhances communication between the care-receiver and their doctors, family members, and caregivers. It manages both personal and medical information, while meeting the care-receiver's needs for privacy and security. At a minimum, the site allows an individual to record both personal and medical history information, link to helpful information, print reports, receive reminder messages about prescription refills and medical appointments.

You are also invited to participate in our caregiving community. We offer a blog and forum to discuss important issues, and to share stories. We also offer a Caregiver's Classified Ads section. This is a good place to buy, sell, barter or trade new and used caregiving products. Also, through the classifieds you can search for a caregiver or get a referral.

www.MeAndMyCaregivers.com

Notes

Notes

Notes